HOW TO PRESENT
AT MEETINGS

Edited by

George M Hall
Professor of Anaesthesia and Intensive Care Medicine
St George's Hospital Medical School, London

© BMJ Books 2001
BMJ Books is an imprint of the BMJ Publishing Group

First published in 2001
by BMJ Books, BMA House, Tavistock Square,
London WC1H 9JR

www.bmjbooks.com

British Library Cataloguing in Publication Data

A catalogue record for this book is available from the British Library

ISBN 0-7279-1572-X

Cover design by BCD Design Ltd, London
Typeset by FiSH Books
Printed and bound by JW Arrowsmith

Contents

Contributors

Martin Godfrey
Vice President of Marketing
Medschool.com
Santa Monica, USA

Angela Hall
Senior Lecturer in Communication Skills
St George's Hospital Medical School
London

George M Hall
Professor of Anaesthesia and Intensive Care Medicine
St George's Hospital Medical School
London

Roger Horton
Professor of Neuropharmacology and Vice Principal
St George's Hospital Medical School
London

Gavin Kenny
Professor of Anaesthesia
University of Glasgow

Sir Alexander Macara
Visiting Professor of Health Studies
University of York, York
Past Chairman
British Medical Association, London

Alan Maryon Davis
Senior Lecturer in Public Health Medicine
King's College, London

Peter McCrorie
Reader in Medical Education
Director of Graduate Entry Programme
St George's Hospital Medical School
London

Mal Morgan
Reader in Anaesthetic Practice
Imperial College School of Medicine
Honorary Consultant Anaesthetist
Hammersmith Hospital
London

Richard Smith
Editor, *British Medical Journal*
London

Preface

Many trainees in medicine, while competent in their specialty, struggle to give a good presentation at a meeting. The aim of this book is to provide a basic framework around which a proficient talk can be built. The content covers not only the essential parts of a presentation; preparation, visual aids and computer-generated slides, but also provides advice on how to sell a message, how to appear on stage and how to deal with questions. All contributors are experienced speakers and provide simple didactic advice. I am grateful for their enthusiastic co-operation.

George M Hall

1 Principles of communication

ANGELA HALL AND PETER McCRORIE

Many readers of this book will have attended conferences and listened to doctors making presentations. Think about these presentations. Which ones were memorable and why?

Communication is, by definition, a two-way process – an interaction. Presentation tends to be one way only, so is there anything at all that we can take from research underlying communication and how people learn, that is of any relevance to the topic of this book? Assuming that the intention of your presentation is to inform your audience, so that something is learned from you, what do we know in general about how people learn?

People learn best when:[1]

- they are motivated
- they recognise their need to learn
- the learning is relevant, in context and matches their needs
- the aims of the learning are clear
- they are actively involved
- a variety of learning methods is used
- it is enjoyable.

Presenting at meetings is not of course just about giving information ("I told them, therefore they know it") but about imparting it in such a way that people understand and take something away from it. Can we draw a parallel with the information-giving process between doctors and patients? There is in fact much evidence from research into medical communication showing that the following behaviours result in the effective transmission of information from doctor to patient.[2]

- Decide on the key information that the patient needs to understand.
- Signpost to the patient what you are going to discuss.
- Find out what the patient knows or understands already.
- Make it manageable – divide it into chunks.
- Use clear, unambiguous language.
- Pace the information so that the patient does not feel overwhelmed.
- Check what the patient has understood.
- Invite questions.

Adopting these behaviours means that, as a doctor, you are doing your best to ensure that your patient both hears and understands what has been said.

What can we take from these two sets of principles that is directly relevant to giving presentations at meetings?

Preparation

Know your audience

Decide what it is about your topic that you want your audience to understand. The presenter is usually in the situation of knowing a lot more about the subject than many of the people in the audience. Find out about your audience. What is their level of knowledge likely to be? How many are likely to be there? The smaller the number, the greater the potential for interaction. Is the language in which you are giving your presentation your audience's first language? Regardless of first language, will your audience have a feel for the technical/medical/scientific terminology with which you are so familiar? Above all, avoid the temptation to try to impart more information than your audience can possibly assimilate. Message – keep it simple.

Don't let yourself get too anxious

Anxiety on the part of either the giver or receiver can act as a barrier to effective communication. Most experienced presenters will tell you that they are always anxious before starting their talk and this does not necessarily get better over time. It is normal and can be advantageous – a certain amount of adrenaline actually makes for a more exciting presentation. Lack of anxiety often results in the presentation appearing a bit flat. On the other hand, too much anxiety is a problem not only for the speaker but also for the audience. An audience can feel embarrassed and show more concern for the state of mind of the speaker than for what is being communicated. Sometimes deep-breathing exercises can help. Most people find that once they get started, anxiety drops to manageable levels. As with an examination, the worst time is just before you turn over the paper.

Rehearse your presentation

An important key to anxiety reduction is to *know* that you are properly prepared. Not only should you be sure about what you are going to say but how long it will take to say it. This means practising your presentation, preferably in front of colleagues whom you trust and who will give you constructive feedback. It is highly unprofessional to over-run and encroach on other speakers' time. A good chairperson will not permit this anyway, with the inevitable result that your talk will be incomplete or rushed at the end. Rehearsal is important.

Prepare prompt cards

What do you take in with you in the form of notes to your presentation? If all you do is read directly from a prepared script, there will be no effective communication with your audience. You might as well have distributed a photocopy of your talk and asked the audience to sit and read it.

Reading also removes any opportunity for eye contact, for judging how the presentation is being received, or for spontaneity. Have you ever laughed at a joke that has been read out to you? A far better solution is to use prompt cards. Prompt cards carry only the key points of your talk. They serve partly as an *aide memoire* and partly as a means of reducing the anxiety of drying up.

Check out the venue and equipment

Arrive at the venue early enough to check out the room size and layout, the location of light switches and the equipment you are intending to use. If you have opted for a PowerPoint presentation, check that the system is compatible with your computer/floppy.

Always bring back-up overhead transparencies – just in case disaster strikes. Check that your slides/overheads are visible from the back of the hall. Be sure you know how to operate the equipment – slide projector/OHP controls, laser pointers, lectern layout, video recorders, etc. The audience will be irritated if you are apparently experimenting with your equipment at the start of your presentation.

Content

Say what you're going to say; say it; then say what you've said

All presentations should have a beginning, a middle, and an end. First, you describe the purpose of the talk and the key areas you will be considering. Second, you deliver the main content of the talk. This should cover:

- why the work was done
- how it was done
- what was found
- what it means.

Finally, you should summarise what you have said in a clear and concise way. Don't worry about repeating yourself. Repetition aids understanding and learning.

Put your talk in context

It is often erroneously assumed that an audience understands the context of a presentation. An example will illustrate this. Try to memorise as many of the following statements as you can.

- A newspaper is better than a magazine.
- A seashore is a better place than the street.
- At first, it is better to run than to walk.
- You may have to try several times.
- It takes some skill but it's easy to learn.
- Even young children can enjoy it.
- Once successful, complications are minimal.
- Birds seldom get too close.
- Rain, however, soaks very fast.

- Too many people doing the same thing can also cause problems.
- One needs lots of room.
- If there are no complications, it can be very peaceful.
- A rock will serve as an anchor.
- If things break loose from it, however, you will not get a second chance.

It's hard, isn't it? Now reread the statements in the knowledge that the title (i.e. the context) of the exercise is "making and flying a kite". This time, you will find it easier to recall the statements. Although this example may seem a little unusual, there is much documented evidence in educational research showing that learners are often not able to relate new knowledge to whatever they already know about a certain subject. Having a context through which new information can be related to existing knowledge results in better memory recall.[3] It is also important to put your presentation into a more general context – how it relates to others speaking in the same session, the meeting or conference theme.

Delivery

Pretend you are on stage

Giving a talk is not unlike being on stage. First impressions matter, so do not shuffle, fidget, mumble, or talk to the projector screen. You do not want the audience to be distracted from what you are saying by how you behave. Remember that your non-verbal communication is as important as the words that you use. Grab the attention of your audience right from the start; you can appeal to their curiosity, tell an anecdote, use a powerful and pertinent quote. Smile and look confident. Speak slowly and clearly and vary your tone of voice. Look around your audience as you talk. Catch their eyes and engage them by being enthusiastic, even passionate, about your subject.

Decide on your mode of delivery

The medium of presentation needs some careful thought. The obvious contenders are slides, overheads and PowerPoint presentations. Which is best for you? With which are you most comfortable? Which is the most impressive? Which best illustrates the material you wish to present? These are questions only you can answer. You must weigh up the pros and cons and make a decision.

Make your visual aids clear and simple

Just as doctors can reinforce the information they give to patients with written materials or simple diagrams or drawings, your visual aids should illuminate or illustrate your words. If you are showing a slide for instance, it is enormously helpful to state what in general it is about as you show it. If your audience needs to read something on your slide or overhead, stay silent for a few seconds. You will be very familiar with your material but do not assume that your audience shares your understanding; for example say what the "x" and "y" axes represent on a graph; explain the key to your histograms. We would probably all like a pound for every slide or overhead that we have been shown in a scientific presentation that is impossible to see or interpret, for which the presenter apologises to the audience. So why show it? Why not make a new slide which summarises the point that the original was attempting to make?

Consider varying the delivery mode

Attention span is limited, especially if your audience is sitting through a series of presentations. In a presentation lasting more than 15–20 minutes, it is worth thinking about switching modes of delivery – for instance, to use a video clip to illuminate a particular point which you wish to drive home. Think about the visual impact of being *shown* an operating technique, for instance, versus a verbal description of it. Or a real patient describing a condition they suffer from, versus your description of what such a patient might say.

Don't go over the top

We have all been to presentations that were dazzling – dual projection, fancy animated PowerPoint slides, videoclips, etc. But have we remembered a thing about the content of these glitzy presentations? Probably not. What is crucial is not to allow the medium to overwhelm the message. It may seem an obvious point, but the greater the number of modes of delivery, the greater the risk of technical failure.

Don't be frightened of questions

What is unpredictable, and invokes much anxiety, is the prospect of being asked difficult or awkward questions at the end. This is dealt with in more detail in Chapter 8, but remember that there will always be questioners who are trying to score points, gain attention, or display knowledge rather than genuinely trying to find out more about your work or ideas. The audience is usually aware of this and will be on your side. If you know that there are areas in your presentation that may confound or compromise some of the evidence that you are presenting, address these in the body of your talk to pre-empt obvious points of attack from questioners. Remember that good research provokes as many questions as it answers and occasionally a member of the audience will ask the question that you had not thought of that will trigger your next research proposal. Doctors should not pretend that they know the answer to a patient's question when they do not. Similarly, admit to your audience if you cannot answer one of its questions, agree to find out the answer and remember to follow it up. You can sometimes engage your audience more actively if you throw the question back.

Look out for non-verbal communication

How you check what the audience has understood from your talk is clearly difficult though not impossible. The questions that you are asked at the end of the talk may give you some insight into the level of comprehension. But what does it mean if no questions are asked at all? What is conveyed to you non-verbally from the audience during your presentation may be just as revealing. Do people look interested or puzzled? How many have gone to sleep? How many are fidgeting or have actually left the room? If you spot any such behaviour, either bring your talk to a conclusion or do something to wake up the audience, such as asking a question or telling an amusing anecdote.

Conclusion

There is real satisfaction to be had from giving a presentation that is well thought out, properly rehearsed, and confidently and enthusiastically delivered. Indeed, anything less indicates lack of respect for your audience and will leave you feeling embarrassed and disinclined ever to repeat the experience. Abraham Lincoln said, memorably: 'If I had six hours to chop down a tree, I should spend the first four hours sharpening the axe'. The message is clear. Your presentation will be great if your preparation has been thorough. Take heart from the experience of most presenters which is that although they may feel very nervous beforehand, once started they actually enjoy the experience. There are few highs to be compared with knowing that your careful preparation paid off and you got it absolutely right.

Summary

- Presentation tends to be a one way communication process

- Prepare your presentation well by understanding your audience, rehearsing your presentation, preparing prompt cards and checking the venue and equipment

- Think of the content: describe the purpose of the talk, deliver the talk and summarise

- The delivery of the presentation is important – think carefully about both verbal and non-verbal communication and visual aids

References

1 Silverman J, Kurtz S, Draper J. *Skills for communicating with patients*. Radcliffe Medical Press, 1998.
2 Knowles M. *The adult learner, a neglected species*. Houston: Gulf Publishing Company, 1990.
3 Schmidt H. Foundations of problem-based learning: some explanatory notes. *Med. Education* 1993; 27:422–32.

2 Preparation of the talk

MAL MORGAN

The medically qualified actor, Richard Leech, stated that lecturing is like acting, in that the object of both is to tell a tale to an audience, but that the former is more difficult because you have to write the script as well. Contrary to popular belief, good lecturers are not born with an innate talent to lecture, although some do have more confidence than others to speak in public; this is not synonymous with being able to deliver a good lecture. However, like everything else, it is a skill that can be learnt, just like inserting a central venous line. It requires practice, discipline and adherence to a reasonably strict set of guidelines.

The two basic tenets of a good lecture are meticulous preparation, which takes time, and rehearsal. How do you go about preparing a lecture?

The invitation

The first time you are invited to lecture will engender a number of emotions, pride, to why me? to sheer terror. It is true to say that there are a minority of people who are quite unable to stand up and talk in front of an audience, and if you are one of these then say so immediately. The organisers of the meeting want and should get a prompt reply. Whether you accept will depend on: (*a*) the subject and whether it is in your area of expertise (if you are an obstetric anaesthetist, do not accept an invitation to talk on "The History of Medieval Welsh Codpieces"); (*b*) whether you have sufficient time to prepare the talk (it always takes longer than you think). It is absolutely essential that you read the invitation carefully to establish the "ground rules" before you accept. Always keep a copy of this letter.

If you have reason to believe that you are not the first choice for this lecture, then do not be put off. Here you have a real opportunity to shine and make a name for yourself. Lectures given under these circumstances can give your career a lot of impetus.

Having accepted, you must now establish from the organisers a number of facts.

Type of meeting

This should be obvious from the invitation, but it isn't always so. Is it a "one off" guest lecture or is it part of a symposium? If the latter, ask for a copy of the programme so that you know who the other speakers are in your session. As the subjects are likely to be similar in your session, it is never a bad idea to contact the other speakers to find out what they are going to cover. Do not be put off if you are told "Oh, I haven't thought about it yet". If it is a research meeting of a society, you are not usually invited, but rather told by someone that you are speaking. These societies usually have strict rules of presentation that must be observed.

Subject

If you are speaking at a symposium there is little leeway with regard to the subject, but if it is a guest lecture, then you can negotiate with the organiser. Establish whether they want a review of the topic, or some of your original research around which you can build up a story, or whether they just want a discussion on future developments. Very often they will leave the entire content to you and, on occasion, allow you to choose whatever subject you like. Under these circumstances you have no excuse whatsoever to deliver a poor lecture.

Timing

Again this should be obvious, but check, and also see if there will be time for questions. It is never acceptable to talk over your allotted time, but no one will ever complain if you finish a little early.

Abstract

Establish at this stage whether an abstract is required for the meeting and if so what is the deadline. As abstracts are often required several months in advance for major meetings, this usually precedes the start of preparation of your lecture and merely indicates that they are of little value. However, if you know an abstract is required, it should be delivered by the deadline (and might even persuade you to start on your talk much earlier); not to do so is unprofessional.

Audience

Basic to the preparation of any lecture is a knowledge of who the audience are likely to be. This gives you some idea of what "level" to pitch the lecture; on the vast majority of occasions of course, these are your peers and therefore there will be no problem. The great mistake is to misjudge your audience, which is not a fault confined to prime ministers. You will leave a very bad impression if you "talk down" to an audience, or on the other hand, "talk over their heads". This is one of the most difficult aspects of lecturing and applies especially if there are lay people present. How to judge this will only come with experience, but a basic rule is not to try to impress the audience but rather to interest them. If you can do this, then they will be impressed, especially if you have been dealing with a difficult and complex topic.

It is also nice to know whether any eminent members of the profession and your specialty are going to be present, that is any "heavies". You should certainly not be put off by this, but in fact should feel proud that they have come to your talk. Contrary to popular belief, they are not there to shoot you down at the end of your talk; they have all been through what you have and the majority are extremely helpful and complimentary. If they think that you might have gone off the track somewhere, they will tell you politely and usually after question time to save embarrassing you. However, as you will certainly have prepared your talk properly, such a situation will not arise.

The number in the audience is irrelevant. You will do exactly the same amount of preparation and rehearsal for an audience of 10 or 1000.

Title

The only thing that an individual sees about a forthcoming lecture is the title, so some thought should be given to making it attractive. A teaching lecture requires a short, didactic title, while an eponymous lecture usually has an obscure title which attracts people out of curiosity if nothing else. Titles for guest lectures should be in plain English and simple. The philosophy of Richard Asher, one of the greatest medical writers, with regard to titles of papers applies just as well to a lecture. Which would attract the greatest audience "A trial of 4,4-diethylhydroxybalderdashic acid in acute choryzal infections" or "A new treatment for the common cold"?

Preparation

How often have you heard a conversation along the lines: "I see you are lecturing at the Royal College on Friday" and the reply "Oh yes, I must get on and do something about that". The latter person is lying. This is just to give a macho impression that this person can prepare a lecture in three or four days; this is impossible, and in reality this person has been preparing it for months. Proper preparation is the basis of a good lecture and, just as a brilliant actor cannot compensate for a poor play, a skilled and experienced lecturer cannot compensate for a poorly prepared talk. It is obvious to the audience if the "spade work" hasn't been done. Unfortunately, there is a tendency for lecturers to "go off" as they get older and the reason for this is usually because they ignore the importance and time required for proper presentation. They have done it so often before that they think they can always do it with the minimum preparation.

A long-retired professor of surgery, and a superb lecturer, once said that in preparing a new lecture, it took one hour's preparation for one minute of lecture; he was not far wrong.

How long before the lecture should you start the preparation? In fact you do so immediately you have accepted the invitation, however far in advance of the talk. Long before you put anything on paper, you start thinking about it and this is a vital part of the preparation. You think about the content during idle moments, on your way into work and on the way home. Something your colleagues say might trigger a thought process about your talk and you might get ideas whilst listening to a talk on a completely different subject, for example on a possible layout for the lecture. If you are wise you should jot these things down so that when you finally sit down to formally prepare the talk you will already have a small dossier on the subject. It is surprising how much useful information you already have towards your talk. Never be afraid to ask the advice of your colleagues on the content and layout of your proposed lecture. They will invariably give you useful and valuable advice.

So, how far in advance do you actually start preparation? The answer, as soon as possible, and would that we were all disciplined enough to do that. The aim should be to finish preparation at least one month before the date, including visual aids. It can then be filed away and looked at two or three times before the talk. There is still time to change things if necessary, although if properly prepared, this will not be necessary.

The actual preparation of the lecture should follow a strict discipline. This is basically the same whether it is a 10-minute or a 50-minute talk.

Collection and selection of data

The first essential is to realise that you cannot cover everything that is known about the subject in one lecture and this particularly applies to the shorter presentations. You will already have given a lot of thought to this and the decision on what to select is entirely yours. You will base your selection on the duration of the talk, remembering that it is unprofessional to over-run your allotted time, and the audience. Even if there are "heavies" in the audience, very few will know as much about the subject as you. Remember that your aim is to interest the audience. It is perfectly acceptable to explain at the beginning of longer talks that you are not going to talk about certain aspects of the subject.

Arrangement of data

You have been asked to talk because you are an expert in the field and therefore you have an immense amount of data on the subject. You have selected what you are going to say and you must now reveal this to the audience in a way which is easy to understand and assimilate.

Introduction

The length of the introduction will depend on the duration of the talk and the complexity of the subject. This can be the most difficult part of the talk and if you can introduce something controversial at this stage, so much the better. Do not be afraid to make the introduction simple, especially if there are lay people present; you do not want to lose the audience at this very early stage. Unless you are naturally amusing, it is wisest to avoid being funny. This applies especially to international meetings even if the same language is spoken in the respective countries.

Main message

The preparation of your talk will have largely taken place in the library, where you are surrounded by reference material, or in your office or at home where you will be surrounded by reprints. Your personal computer will have undoubtedly played some part in your preparation, but you may not have many journals on line. It is imperative that you read all the papers to which you refer and not just the summaries. When you have collated all your data, you should write the lecture (some will prefer a word processor) in the order in which you are going to give the talk. Always keep all the references that you have used.

When it comes to delivering the main message, then do so in a logical sequence, using plain English, and giving your supporting evidence. Take the trouble to explain your visual aids, which the audience are seeing for the first time.

Conclusions

At the end of your talk the audience will expect relevant conclusions and it is also sensible to make some suggestions as to where the future lies, if applicable. Remember that if your title asked a question, then the audience have a right to expect an answer.

When you have written the talk you should now make the appropriate visual aids, having already established with the organisers what equipment is available. The lecture and visual aids are then filed. Never throw them away; you never know if they will be useful again.

Rehearsal

This is absolutely mandatory. The rationale behind a rehearsal is:

- to time the lecture, especially the shorter ones
- to assess the technique of delivery, where annoying mannerisms can be spotted and removed
- to anticipate questions
- to give confidence to the speaker.

For ten-minute talks to research societies, the rehearsal should be in front of your colleagues, which is never easy. This should be done a minimum of two weeks in advance so that there is still time to correct slides and iron out flaws in your delivery technique. For the longer talks you should sit with your manuscript and visual aids and go through the talk and slides and time how long it takes. You should do this several times before your talk and you should do it every time you are going to lecture, even if it is the same talk. When rehearsing in this way, always go through the slides as you would at the actual presentation.

Presentation

You are going to be nervous when you stand up in front of an audience to talk, particularly the first time. Although the more experienced lecturers may not give this impression, you can guarantee that there will be a degree of apprehension. Under no circumstances should you resort to pharmacological help to allay this apprehension. It might get less with time, but it will never entirely disappear.

Lectures should not be read. It gives the impression that you don't know your subject and also keeps your head down and encourages you to mumble. Your head must be up, talking to the back row and, in order to do this, you must know and have learned what to say. Use your visual aids as prompts. Turn to them to refresh yourself as to the next point, then turn back to talk to the audience. This means you must learn what you are going to say; actors do.

The only reason why people want to read the manuscript is because they are frightened they might forget to say something. This is totally irrelevant because nobody in the audience would know you were going to say it anyway. If you do suddenly remember that you were going to say something five minutes ago, ignore it; do not go back to it. This does not mean that you shouldn't have the full script available, and even refer to it very briefly from time to time, but the professional doesn't need one.

Visual aids

The most important thing to remember about visual aids is that they are aids. Very clever things can be done with them these days, but they must not be allowed to take over. Superb visual aids cannot compensate for poor content and delivery.

The vast majority of talks involve slides or PowerPoint projection. Whatever you use, some basic points apply:

- Give the impression that you know your slides, so be confident and know what is coming next.
- Use all the information that is on the slide, or it shouldn't be there.
- Disclose the information progressively.
- Never go back, rather use two slides.
- Do not use full sentences.
- Do not read everything that is on the slides
- Never flash through slides.
- Do not leave slides up when you have finished talking about them; arrange your lecture so that this doesn't happen.
- Do not overcrowd slides; use more than one.
- Never borrow slides; always make your own.

So remember, lectures take time to prepare and if your preparation has been meticulous and you have rehearsed your talk with colleagues and sought their advice, the lecture really won't be a problem.

Summary

- The key to a good lecture is preparation and rehearsal
- Check the content of the meeting at which you are going to talk, the subject and timing
- Understand the audience in order to select the right level at which to pitch your presentation
- Think carefully about the title and the content of your talk
- Select and arrange information according to the audience and time given
- Rehearsal is mandatory

3 The three talks

MAL MORGAN

Hospital medical practice would be regarded as strange by many people and particularly the treatment of emergency cases. The latter present many more problems than routine cases, yet they are largely cared for by the junior members of staff. The same applies to lecturing in the medical world. The shorter the talk, the harder it is to prepare and deliver. Yet the five-minute talk is usually delegated to house officers or senior house officers, the 10–15 minute talk to specialist registrars, while the 45-minute lectures are the province of consultants.

There are no rules about lecturing, but a format has developed which has stood the test of time and it works. Talks of different lengths require slightly different techniques, but the general principles are the same.

General principles

- You are in a conservative profession so dress accordingly. A slipshod appearance equates to slipshod work in the minds of the audience.
- Never start a lecture with a slide. You are frightened because everyone is staring at you. Stare back, moving your head slightly from side to side. The audience have a right to see who is talking to them.
- After your introduction and the first slide comes up, the lights go down and should not come on again until you have finished. Conclude with the lights on.
- Speak to the audience, only turning to your slides to ensure that it is the correct one or to illustrate some point.
- Stand still when you are talking. Actors always like to deliver their lines whilst stationary.

- Talk at your normal rate. Radio newsreaders talk at about 120–133 words per minute. The rate of speaking of five subjects experienced in presenting papers and difficult material clearly varies from 106–158 words per minute. Never try to talk more quickly to get more information across.
- At international meetings it is a courtesy to talk more slowly. If there is simultaneous translation, provide a copy of exactly what you are going to say. As the spoken word is different from the written word, it will read terribly but translate perfectly.
- Do not try to be funny unless you are a natural, and smutty stories are strictly forbidden; you will always offend someone.
- When talking, punctuation is replaced by changes in the tone of voice, pauses and gestures. A monotonous voice with few pauses will guarantee that some members of audience will go to sleep.
- Visual aids are an integral part of any good lecture and very few people have the gift of holding an audience's attention without them.

  (*a*) Blackboard and chalk (whiteboard and pencil, etc). This still has a place and can't be beaten when teaching small groups. The author, however, has seen Professor Patrick Wall hold an audience of 400 enthralled using a blackboard. Flip charts are dreadful.

  (*b*) Overhead projector. Again usually used as a teaching aid and has the advantage that the lecturer can face the audience at all times. The overheads require as much preparation and care as slides.

  (*c*) Slides. These have been the mainstay of lectures for many years. The requirements for good slides are found in Chapter 4, but remember they require a projector and possibly a projectionist. Always check whether the projector is automatic, or not, well in advance. Slide projectors do go wrong and if you are using dual projection, which can be very effective, then you double the likelihood of problems. An additional problem has crept in of late, namely that of back projection. This means that the slides have to be inserted into the carousel completely differently from forward projection. You must check this and go through all your slides to see that they are correctly inserted, otherwise your talk can deteriorate into a complete shambles.

  (*d*) PowerPoint. This is gradually taking over from slides and, if used correctly, is extremely effective. But computer-generated slides can and do go wrong, much more frequently than slides. Your disc must be compatible with the hardware that is in use and you should have been told by the organisers what equipment they have. The biggest danger is that you are using the latest software, but the organisers are not. Great people (and the audience) have been embarrassed by having to wait 15 minutes or more before they have functioning visual aids. At the moment, the wise lecturer always takes slides along as back-up.

(e) Videos (films are a thing of the past) are only rarely needed to complement a lecture and, when indicated, can be very worthwhile. However, they can go wrong. A good projectionist is essential if things are to go smoothly and you should talk to them will in advance and have a practice run-through. The video must be switched off immediately after your point has been made.

- Rehearse, rehearse, rehearse.

Day of the lecture

Despite your nerves, you must check a number of points when you arrive.

The chairman

Seek out the chairman and introduce yourself. You might know him/her, but he/she is unlikely to know you, especially when you are starting out in your career. Chairmen get nervous too and want to know that their speakers are present.

The lectern

Look at this beforehand and familiarise yourself with the layout. Lecterns can vary considerably from being very simple to resembling a Boeing 747 cockpit. Ensure that you know how to call up your slides, especially the first one. Check whether you can focus the slides yourself and whether you, or the projectionist, controls the lights. A good chairman will know what to do, but chairmen vary as well.

The microphone

The best are pinned to your clothing, which allows you some movement whilst talking without the sound level varying; fixed microphones have the disadvantage that you have to ensure that you are talking into it at roughly the same distance all the time, even when you turn to your slides. This is where overhead and PowerPoint projections have advantages. When you stand up on the podium, pin the microphone on yourself and do it quickly.

The pointer

This will either be something elongated (billiard cues are favourites) or, more often nowadays, a laser pointer (where the battery is usually on the verge of failing – check beforehand). Whatever the pointer, the technique of using it is the same. Always point to the aspect under discussion so that it is clear to the audience. Complicated illustrations can require a lot of "pointing". If you are worried about a tremor when using a laser pointer, then hold it in both hands whilst steadying yourself by leaning on the lectern. Remember to switch off the laser after making your point, as it is potentially dangerous to leave it on when you turn to face the audience as eyes can be damaged.

Once you are satisfied with all the above points, check them again. The classic mistake with slides is to find that the last and "crunch" one has been left in the projector back home where you have been rehearsing.

The five-minute talk

These are usually the province of the most junior members of the profession, who are told by their seniors that they are going to do it, and they have no say in the matter. Furthermore, the notice is usually short and you will be lucky if you have two weeks; 24 hours is not unusual.

Such talks usually involve case reports, or some aspect of an interesting case, with a mini review of the salient features. The fact that the time for preparation is short must not be used as an excuse for a slipshod presentation. Presenting all the important features in five minutes is not easy and the use of visual aids will be limited.

- It is not necessary to prepare slides or a PowerPoint presentation for this sort of talk.
- Blackboard and chalk will slow you down and is not ideal.
- This is where the overhead projector comes into its own.

The overheads must be prepared in advance but do not overcrowd them. It is quite permissible to write them rather than get them typed. Make sure that they are in order and that they do not stick together. There must be a flat surface on which to place the overhead once it has been used and another on the other side of the projector for the ones you are going to use; *do not confuse them*. Practice with the overheads before your presentation so that delays are avoided. It is embarrassing to see people fumbling with their overheads during the talk.

Some people like to reveal the points on the overheads one by one by covering them up with a piece of paper. This is not necessary and is never done with slides

- If you are going to show radiographs make sure that you have them in your possession (there is a great tendency for them to go missing) and that you have a functioning viewing box.
- You might be presenting a patient; remember to explain everything to him/her. You must preserve their dignity at all times.
- Even though the notice might have been short, you should try to find time to rehearse; you can always find a colleague willing to spare a few minutes. Over-running on such a short talk is indefensible.

The 15-minute talk

Such talks are usually the remit of more senior members of the trainee staff such as specialist registrars. You might be told you are doing this or be chosen by agreement.

Talks of this duration are usually a research presentation to a society and you will have been one of the workers involved in the project. This work might have been going on for a year or more. It would be unfair not to admit that these presentations cause more angst and stress than any other. Senior academic members of the profession will be present and you will be terrified that you might make a fool of yourself. But remember that you have been working in the field for some time and you will know the subject intimately. There will be very few people present with such detailed knowledge. Conversely, of course, you are going to have to present your information in such a way that it is going to interest the vast majority of the audience who will only have a passing acquaintance with the subject. Putting facts that you know well to a general audience requires considerable skill.

There are a number of points to bear in mind when you have been chosen to give such a talk:

- A research society will probably have rules, for example nothing must be read, know these rules.
- You have been chosen to present the results of research work that might have been going on for a year or more and involved several collaborators. You must not let them or yourself, down, so preparation must be meticulous.
- You cannot get a year or more's research work into 15 minutes. Selection of data is therefore vital and you must decide with your co-workers what you want to get across; this will probably be only one major point. Do not try to give more information than anyone can assimilate in 15 minutes.
- The introduction must be brief and state why you did the work. Give enough information so that the audience knows how you did your measurements; things can be expanded during questions. In such a short talk you should use only your own original material and should not show slides of other people's work to illustrate a point.
- Do not be tempted to use too many slides. For a ten-minute talk, eight will be the maximum and six are preferable.
- Speak at your normal rate. Do not be tempted to show an extra slide or two by talking more quickly. This never works.
- Rehearsal in front of colleagues is mandatory, including a final dress rehearsal. This is often stressful and you might feel foolish, but it must be done, and done in the way in which you are going to deliver your definitive talk. Rehearse as often as is necessary to get it perfect.

The 45-minute talk

These talks are usually given by the more senior members of the profession and are usually by invitation. The first time you are asked, the organisers might well be "just trying you out". A successful talk will usually mean that you get further invitations as word soon gets around; eventually you will become an established lecturer.

Once established, never lower your standards. Don't become blasé and think you can always deliver a good lecture. Preparation is everything and if you let this slip (usually because you are in a hurry), then a poor talk will result. Make sure that it is never you they are talking about when you hear "he used to be a good lecturer".

There are several types of 45-minute talks.

The teaching lecture

Above all, be enthusiastic and show the audience that you know the topic. Put yourself in the position of one of the audience and ask what you want from a teaching lecture.

- The subject should be presented in a logical order, with clear headings and some discussion after each. Additional visual aids can be used to illustrate a point.
- Do not try to get too much in one lecture. If it is impossible to get over all the points, either decline the invitation or ask for two lecturers.
- Deliver the lecture at such a speed that notes can be taken.
- Use clear visual aids. A big advantage of blackboard and chalk is that you can build up a topic in front of an audience and it slows you down.

Keep the lecture up to date by reviewing it in your office from time to time. You should not be giving the same talk in 10 years' time – there will have been some changes.

At a symposium

You will have been invited to do this because you are well known in the field. Again, selection of data is critical and it is important to judge your audience correctly, which you should have done in advance. The subject of this type of lecture is usually chosen for you.

The guest lecture

Here the field is yours and you should establish from your host a rough idea of the subject matter. You have no excuse for not preparing a talk such as this properly, particularly if the subject is left entirely up to you.

The eponymous lecture

Usually given by the good and the great at the culmination of their career. These talks usually attract the most senior members of the specialty and frequently those from other disciplines; lay people often attend.

It is customary to say something about the person whose name is attached to the lecture, remembering that members of the family may be present. If possible try to say something that leads into the substance of your talk. These days, the latter does not have to relate to the interest of the person whose name you are honouring. Occasionally, eponymous lectures are given at the start of your career and this can certainly help your advancement "up the ladder".

Is it worth it?

This is a question often asked by those who have gone through the problems of preparing and delivering talks at important meetings. Some do not think it worthwhile and never present again. However, there is no doubt that the feelings engendered after you have delivered a well received lecture are extremely pleasant and many revel in being the centre of attention in the immediate post-lecture period.

On the other hand, you might like to read the paper by Taggart and colleagues before answering the question.

Summary

- Talks of different lengths require slightly different techniques but the general principles are the same
- Use an overhead projector for a five minute talk
- For a fifteen minute talk information must be brief and to the point. Six to eight slides will suffice
- There are several types of 'forty-five minute' talks: the teaching lecture, at a symposium, the guest lecture and the eponymous lecture and you should prepare for each type accordingly

Further reading

Taggart P, Carruthers M, Somerville W. Electrocardiogram, plasma catecholamines and lipids, and their modification by oxprenalol when speaking before an audience. *Lancet* 1973:2 341–6

Whitwam JG. Spoken communication. *Br J Anaesth* 1970: **42**:768–78.

4 Visual aids

GEORGE M HALL

Visual aids are essential in medical presentations and much thought must be given to this part of the talk. Very few speakers can hold the attention of the audience for more than a few minutes without using slides. It is very difficult to convey information clearly without visual aids. An excellent lecture can be ruined by inappropriate and illegible slides, or technical problems when the local equipment refuses to project your version of PowerPoint. Good visual aids always enhance a presentation and their skillful use should be learnt at an early stage in a medical career. The basic aids are:

- board and coloured pens
- flipchart
- overhead projector and acetate sheets
- video
- slides.

The most commonly used visual aid is the slide, either prepared before the talk or projected from a PC. However, the other methods merit brief comments.

Board and coloured pens

The forerunner of this technique was the blackboard and coloured chalks. Unless you really wanted to be an artist or graphic designer and have the necessary talent, do not bother to consider this as a possible medium. I have seen brilliant displays with coloured pens by anatomists as they have slowly and patiently explained the development of an organ but this is a dying art and far beyond mere mortals. Remember that most people cannot write on a board in a straight line.

Flipcharts

These are best kept for those in medical management who wish to scribble two or three words on a large piece of paper before hurriedly covering it lest their illogical thinking is obvious to the audience. However, if you belong to the "I love clinical governance" minority sect you may find a flipchart helpful in confusing the audience.

Overhead projector

The acetate sheets needed for this visual aid must be prepared just as rigorously as slides (see below). With the introduction of PowerPoint the overhead projector has become less popular but it is still useful for a brief, 5–10 minute, presentation.

Videos

Videos are occasionally valuable in demonstrating a new practical technique. It is essential to obtain expert help, often from the university or medical school audio-visual department, to ensure that the video is of high quality. Do not assume that, because you can film the family barbecue on a damp Sunday in Sidcup, you are a budding Scorcese. A good medical video needs to be made by a skilled professional.

Slides

The guidelines for the preparation of slides have been well known for many years and yet basic mistakes continue to be made. If you are a novice, seek help and advice from senior colleagues who are recognised for their presentational skills. In many medical schools the audio-visual department is very willing to give practical advice and even show examples of how not to do it. Remember that visual aids are used to add to the content of the talk and should not distract with garish colours, silly logos, and sound effects suitable for children's television. The ready availability of computer software packages such as PowerPoint (Microsoft) means that it is easy to prepare clear slides. However, it is also possible to make a visual mess with this programme (see Chapter 5). Guidelines for slide preparation can be considered under the following headings:

- general format
- text
- figures
- tables.

General format (see Box **4.1**)

The key principle to remember is "the fewer slides the better". A problem with using programmes, such as PowerPoint, is that it is easy to present too many slides, so that the impression left with the audience may be literally that of a "moving picture show" as slides flash by. The absolute maximum number of slides is one for each minute of the talk and a more sensible rate of projection is six slides per ten minutes of talk.

Box 4.1 General format

- The fewer slides the better
- Plain uncluttered slides are easier to read
- Choose colours carefully, avoid two dark colours
- Keep to horizontal orientation
- Use the same format for all slides – colour combinations, typeface and layout

---

A plain uncluttered appearance of the slide is necessary to emphasise the content. Avoid logos: most of the audience are not interested in where you work and know that they are attending the Third International Congress on Equine Euthanasia. Avoid frilly edges to the slide: the audience will think that you are a dress designer or worse; and avoid moving images, unless you want to ensure that the slide is not read.

The choice of colours is of great importance. It is traditional to use a light colour on a dark background, such as yellow or white on a blue background and many different shades of these colours are available. Although out of favour at present, a dark text on a light background works well. The original technique was to use black lettering on white (a positive slide) and this is useful in situations in which the light in the lecture room can only be partially dimmed. A more modern equivalent is to use black on a light grey background. Never use dark colours on a dark background – red on a dark blue background is a favourite combination and it is hopeless. Remember that the road signs in the UK are yellow on a dark green background or black on a white background because these combinations have been found to be the easiest to read. If you are unsure about the colours to use, let the Department of Transport be your guide.

If possible, try to keep all the slides in a horizontal orientation. Standard slides are mounted in 50·8 mm (2 in) square mounts, but produce rectangular images. Most slides are shown with the long axis horizontally and the short axis vertically (approximate proportions of 3:2). If you use slides with a vertical layout then you run the risk of losing the top or bottom of the slide as some lecture theatres cannot deal with this orientation. It is very irritating to see some of the slide projected on to the ceiling or floor.

Finally, use the same format for all the slides, that is, the same colour combinations, typeface, layout, etc. If you want your presentation to be taken as a coherent talk then your slides must reflect this and be consistent. Do not insult the audience by presenting them with a jumble of slides, sometimes known as "pick-and-mix" slides, which you have obviously used before for many different talks. Instead of listening to the content of the lecture, the audience will be wondering on whom you last inflicted that dreadful, rainbow-coloured, illegible slide.

Text (see Box **4.2**)

The most common mistake is to try to present too much information on a single slide. Never use more than eight lines per slide and if at all possible stop at six lines. If necessary, divide the content between two slides rather than cram in extra lines. This is a fundamental rule of slide preparation and must never be broken.

Do not write in complete sentences, unless they are very short, just give the key words in a single line. It is always preferable to keep to a single line for each point that you are making: you lose impact by using two or, even worse, three lines. Select a clear uncluttered typeface that can be read easily, scan some of the newspapers to gain ideas about those typefaces that can be read best at a distance. Avoid upper case text (capital letters) as this is more difficult to read quickly than lower case text. If you wish to emphasise a point, underline the relevant word; a different typeface occasionally works but can distract from the rest of the slide. The text should be aligned from the left, with the right margin left unjustified.

Box 4.2 Text

- Six lines preferable, never more than eight
- Give key words on a single line
- Select clear typeface
- Avoid upper case text (capital letters)
- Align text from left, right margin is not justified

The golden rule is to keep the slides simple and avoid detail. If you have to explain the layout of a slide to the audience then you have failed.

Figures (see Box **4.3**)

There is considerable scope for making a mess when drawing figures for slides. The same general principles apply to figures as to the text: the colour combinations must be consistent throughout the presentation and it is essential to avoid overcrowding the figures. Because the editor of a journal insisted that you combine four small graphs into a single figure does not mean that you should inflict the same layout on the audience. The decision of the editor was based on the need to save space in the journal; your objective is completely different – that of imparting information with clear, unambiguous slides, so the rule is one graph for one slide.

Complicated pie charts often look impressive in publications but are not suitable for slides because it is difficult for the audience to assimilate the information rapidly. It is preferable to use different symbols for different lines on a graph rather than different colours.

Box 4.3 Figures

- One graph for each slide
- Use different symbols for different lines and not different colours
- Give indication of variability, if possible
- Label axes horizontally
- Avoid 3-D images

This avoids confusion where lines cross or disappear into overlapping mean values. Although it seems instinctive to consider different colours for different lines, this only works if the lines are well separated. If possible try to give an indication of the variability of the data but look carefully to be certain that this does not make the slide messy and detract from the message. If necessary, you simply tell the audience that the data on the variability of the results are available and that they will have to trust your statistical analysis for the presentation. All labels should be written horizontally, abbreviated if necessary – unless you like inducing neck injuries in the audience – and should be self-explanatory. You undoubtedly remember whom groups 1-4 were, but most of the audience forgot 15 minutes ago, so label them appropriately – for example: sober, mildly drunk, very drunk, and members of college council. Avoid whizzy 3-D options: in most instances they add nothing to the presentation and just tell the audience that you are an anorak who reads the software manual.

Tables (see Box 4.4)

Tables should only be used in slides if they are very simple, as it takes much longer to read a table than it does to "read" the same information presented as a figure. Again the same basic principles

Box 4.4 Tables

- Tables must be very simple
- Tables used for publication are usually not suitable for presentation
- Alignment of columns is essential
- Use explicit labels and give units of measurement

apply: consistent colour combinations, a simple typeface and a clear layout. Alignment of the columns is essential in a table, otherwise the eye is drawn inevitably to the misalignment and obvious kinks. As for figures, use explicit labels and give units of measurement. It is almost always true to say that a table prepared for publication is totally unsuitable for presentation as a slide. For example, Tables 4.1 and 4.2 are taken from recent issues of the BMJ and must never be used as a slide. There is far too much information and most of it will be illegible when viewed from a distance. In marked contrast, tables suitable for slides are shown in Tables 4.3 and 4.4.

Table 4.1 24 Hour means (SDs) for air pollutants (μg/m³ except PM₁₀ – ppb) and daily incidence of wheezy cases and controls

	Spring	Summer	Autumn	Winter	All seasons
Pollutant					
Ozone	46.3 (16.7)***	40.6 (13.3)***	22.0 (15.4)	22.3 (15.9)	32.7 (18.8)
SO₂	13.6 (11.5)***	14.7 (14.3)***	14.7 (13.4)	27.7 (24.3)	17.7 (17.5)
NO₂	41.7 (19.1)*	37.8 (14.4)***	46.0 (17.6)***	48.7 (17.4)	43.6 (17.6)
PM₁₀	23.5 (11.6)***	23.8 (10.8)***	19.7 (10.7)***	32.2 (20.1)	24.9 (14.6)
Benzene	2.54 (1.24)**	2.59 (1.33)	5.08 (4.22)	4.08 (2.56)	3.57 (2.83)
1,3-Butadiene	0.86 (0.55)**	1.02 (0.74)	1.82 (2.01)	1.33 (1.34)	1.26 (1.34)
cis-2-Butene	0.19 (0.09)	0.22 (0.10)	0.47 (0.46)**	0.31 (0.30)	0.30 (0.30)
n-Butane	6.12 (3.71)	6.39 (3.57)	13.00 (11.65)**	9.14 (7.53)	8.65 (7.85)
tr-2-Butene	0.40 (0.13)	0.43 (0.16)	0.77 (0.64)**	0.54 (0.42)	0.53 (0.42)
Ethene	5.27 (2.66)***	5.49 (2.82)***	11.68 (10.00)	10.80 (7.58)	8.29 (7.16)
Ethylbenzene	1.36 (0.67)*	1.44 (0.76)	3.18 (2.85)**	2.17 (1.63)	2.06 (1.89)
Ethyne	3.48 (1.92)**	3.18 (1.66)***	7.08 (6.24)	5.63 (2.68)	4.82 (3.94)
n-Heptane	0.30 (0.15)***	0.30 (0.15)***	0.63 (0.55)	0.52 (0.37)	0.44 (0.37)
n-Hexane	0.69 (0.47)**	0.76 (0.44)**	1.23 (1.04)	1.11 (0.85)	0.94 (0.77)
m+p-Xylene	3.36 (1.74)*	3.62 (2.02)	8.07 (7.31)***	5.29 (4.22)	5.14 (4.86)
o-Xylene	1.38 (0.74)*	1.31 (0.64)*	3.20 (2.99)**	2.23 (1.71)	2.06 (1.95)
cis-2-Pentene	0.14 (0.07)	0.17 (0.99)	0.38 (0.20)***	0.22 (0.20)	0.22 (0.23)
iso-Pentane	6.59 (3.94)	7.67 (4.27)	11.93 (10.86)***	7.56 (7.30)	8.44 (7.41)
trans-2-Pentene	0.23 (0.13)	0.32 (0.19)	0.69 (0.66)***	0.40 (0.38)	0.41 (0.43)
me-Pentane	2.70 (1.47)*	2.93 (1.58)	5.47 (5.17)*	4.12 (3.56)	3.80 (3.48)
n-Pentane	1.32 (0.77)*	1.58 (0.91)	2.61 (2.19)**	1.79 (1.35)	1.82 (1.49)
Toluene	6.37 (3.27)*	6.92 (3.57)	14.00 (12.63)**	9.76 (7.99)	9.26 (8.39)
Ethane	5.15 (2.24)***	3.83 (1.76)***	6.69 (5.14)	7.88 (3.54)	5.88 (3.74)
Propane	2.36 (1.31)***	1.95 (0.99)***	4.02 (3.13)	4.58 (2.27)	3.22 (2.36)
Isoprene	0.26 (0.20)	0.60 (0.31)***	0.48 (0.41)**	0.30 (0.26)	0.41 (0.33)
Average HC	2.45 (1.19)*	2.40 (1.13)*	5.05 (4.25)*	3.75 (2.60)	3.47 (2.86)
Incidence:					
All cases	3.2 (1.9)**	3.2 (2.8)**	5.1 (2.7)	4.5 (2.5)	4.0 (2.6)
Cases <2 years	2.0 (1.0)***	0.8 (1.1)***	2.3 (1.8)	2.0 (1.7)	1.6 (1.6)
Cases >2 years	2.1 (1.5)	2.3 (2.2)	2.8 (1.8)	2.5 (1.9)	2.4 (1.9)
All controls	63.5 (9.8)***	59.5 (10.1)	56.8 (9.9)	56.5 (9.2)	59.1 (10.1)

*p<0.05; **p<0.01;***p<0.001 v winter season.
SO₂=sulphur dioxide; NO₂=nitrogen dioxide; PM₁₀=small particulates with diameter <10 μm; Average HC=average of all 21 hydrocarbons.

Table 4.2 Estimated 8 hour TWA exposures to MBT and its derivative by job and department title and by calendar period*

			Applied to earlier periods					
Department	Department code	Jobs	1955–60	1961–67	1968–77	1978–80	1981–81	1982–85
MBT solution	82936	Autoclave operator, dissolver bath operator, dayman	1.75	1.75	1.75	0.50	0.50	0.50
Bantex or Thiotax	99909	Centrifuge mill operator	4.25	4.25	4.25	1.75	1.75	1.75
"	"	Day bagging operator	4.25	4.25	4.25	4.25	0.88	0.88
"	"	Packing or precipitator operator, flexible operator	1.75	1.75	1.75	1.75	1.75	0.0
Pelleting	99905	Pellet operator	0.0	11.70	11.70	3.83	3.83	1.75
"	"	Day pack operator	0.0	11.70	11.70	2.33	2.33	1.75
Milling and blending	99980	Blending operator	1.95	1.95	1.95	0.64	3.24	3.24
Thiofide	82957	Senior operator, flexible operator	2.25	2.25	2.25	2.25	2.25	0.85
"	"	Bag flake operator, dayman	8.50	8.50	6.00	6.00	6.00	0.85
Thiurams	99970	Filtrate pellet operator	0.0	0.0	2.13	2.13	0.0	0.0
"	"	Dayman	0.0	0.0	6.50	6.50	0.0	0.0
All others	—	—	0.0	0.0	0.0	0.0	0.0	0.0

*The precision suggested by two places of decimals is spurious and should be ignored.

Table 4.3 Definitions

Knowledge	Specific information about a subject
Experience	Direct personal participation or observation
Competence	The condition of being capable; ability; the state of being legally competent or qualified

Table 4.4 Distribution of responses by country

Country	Respondents (n)	Country	Respondents (n)
Austria	2	Latvia	1
Belgium	3	Lithuania	2
Bulgaria	2	Norway	4
Czech Republic	6	Portugal	4
Denmark	2	Russia	1

When all the slides have been prepared, go to a lecture theatre with a colleague and project them. Check very carefully for mistakes, they occur commonly, and are more likely to be spotted by a colleague who has not seen the material before. Your colleague should sit in the back row of the lecture theatre to ensure that all the information can be seen easily. If it cannot, then you have to change the slide. It is sometimes hard to admit that your favourite slide is less than perfect, but it is important to find out well before the presentation. When all the slides are correct then you can start to go through the talk. As you rehearse check that the slides fulfil the basic functions list on page 16 to ensure that they develop a coherent story.

After that you are nearly ready for the presentation. There is still the small matter of rehearsal, rehearsal, and, when you think that the talk is polished, even more rehearsal.

Summary

- Visual aids are essential when giving medical presentations
- Only use board and coloured pens if you have the necessary talent; flipcharts are also not encouraged
- Videos are occasionally valuable in demonstrating a new practical technique
- Slides are the most common form of visual aid used, especially in PowerPoint
- Remember that the fewer slides used the better, keep them simple and make figures and tables easy to understand

5 Computer-generated slides: how to make a mess with PowerPoint

GAVIN KENNY

You have been asked to present the essence of your life's work to date, to give a description of the last patient you treated who exhibited some rare form of eruption, or to summarise and explain the item which caught your tutor's eye in the most recent copy of a journal. How do you start to make a mess of it with PowerPoint? It is important to remember that if you do not have good data, then your audio-visual aids must be outstanding. People will then remember how you faded your slides one into another or the extraordinary way you included a video clip of the Professor of Surgery actually performing an operation.

The most important thing to remember is that you will probably know more about the subject you are presenting than 99% of your audience. However, it is important to be able to identify the remaining 1% correctly so that you agree with their questions before answering them.

Basic requirements

To confuse your audience, you should have no plan whatsoever to your presentation. You should adopt a rambling approach, springing one irrelevant item after another on your initially surprised, then bored and finally, frankly rebellious audience. An alternative approach is to provide a clear, simple presentation where everything that you want the audience to remember particularly is sign-posted clearly. You then adopt the mantle of an author where you have a "story line" along which you guide your audience to understand and marvel at the simple, clear concepts which you have placed before them.

To irritate an audience you should ramble on without regard to time and, ideally, when the chairman warns you that your time is most definitely up, you should show your final ten concluding slides. The best way to deal with this is for the chairman to switch off your microphone and slowly increase the volume of Beethoven's Ninth Symphony on the auditorium speakers. Even with the best audio-visual aids, it is impossible to compete with this.

What medium?

Overhead transparencies are a reliable medium in that you can hold them in your hand. They are quick to produce and you can use PowerPoint to give a wide range of formats and colours. An overhead projector will usually be available but it is really only suitable for a small audience because of the relatively limited power of its systems.

Thirty-five millimetre slides have been the standard medium used throughout the world. They are now produced usually with systems like PowerPoint and you also can hold them in your hand. Most venues where you are asked to present a paper or lecture will have a 35 mm slide projector. However, sometimes these projectors are less than reliable: slides can jam in them, refuse to change to the next, jump two slides at a time or the bulb can blow up and there is no spare. These 35 mm slides are relatively cheap to produce but, increasingly, medical illustration departments are now charging a considerable sum per slide. The cost of a complete presentation can easily be over £100, so there is a tendency to leave slides imperfect. There are also some things about your presentation and slides which you can only really find out when using them to give your talk. It may be that when you show a particular slide, you only realise then that it does not clarify the process which had seemed so simple when you produced that slide. It can take considerable effort to ensure that all of these small or large faults are removed before using these slides again.

A full PowerPoint presentation is a flexible medium in which you can make changes up to, and sometimes even during, the presentation. There is no cost in changing slides which means that it is very simple to get your presentation correct. In addition, there is a choice of different text build, dynamic slide change and the possibility to incorporate graphics and videos. Suitable PC projectors are now available almost universally in most countries and have a standardised connection from the computer. The PC projection system is described by its resolution so that now the lowest acceptable is an SVGA resolution of 800 x 600 pixels, while XGA, which is 1024 x 768 pixels, is rapidly becoming the standard. Older VGA systems with a resolution of 600 x 480 pixels can be used, but are much less satisfactory.

There are special software systems, such as those supplied with some projectors, which will help in the running of a PowerPoint presentation. They offer features such as smoothing the "jaggy" edges of text and allowing you to rapidly select the correct screen display resolution for the PC projector you are using. They can also automatically disable any power-saving features on a computer so that the screen does not suddenly go blank as you make your most important point to the audience.

Always check that the mains power is on

If you are running your presentation from the battery of a laptop computer, the chances are that it will fail half-way through your presentation. Always check that the mains power is actually getting into your laptop. Frequently, this requires the power switch at the wall to be moved to the "on" position.

The entire PowerPoint presentation depends on complex and delicate magneto-mechanical components. Hard disks will crash at some point and it is absolutely essential to ensure adequate back-up of your presentation material – otherwise you may as well have stayed at home. The area of back-up medium is changing constantly but it could range from a simple floppy disk, if your presentation is less than 1·4 megabytes, up to a CD-ROM if you include graphics or video clips. The really concerned, or paranoid, PowerPoint presenter will travel with two laptops and a CD-ROM of their entire slide collection, as well as a back-up hard disk. There is little worse than arriving to give your presentation clutching your Zip disk to then find out that the computer you were planning to use only has a CD-ROM capability.

Slide layout

PowerPoint offers the presenter with an almost infinite number of possibilities to customise the layout of his or her presentation. This is an advantage if you have an innate sense of colour, form and balance but may lead to bizarre combinations and effects if you are a typical doctor. Using one of the standard presentation templates may be a safer option in the first instance. There are a few simple rules such as using a uniform font per slide with appropriate font sizes. The selection of bold text with shadowing can often enhance the legibility of text and there should be an appropriate number of text lines and points to be made with each slide. It is better to use several slides to get your points across rather than cram everything on to one single slide (see Boxes 5.1 and 5.2)

Box 5.1 Poor text layout

This is what can happen if the text is made too small so that considerable amounts of data can be placed on a single slide and the maximum amount of information can then be provided

The effect may be viewable from the front row – just, or with a telescope from the back of the hall

There is little point in attempting to cram so much information into one slide – better to space out the text on to several slides and then the audience will be able to see and hopefully understand exactly what you want

This is especially the case when trying to fit excessive data into a table

There should be no need to apologise for slides unless they are burned by the projector bulb

---

Box 5.2 Good text layout

- Use "bold" and "shadowing" on the text
- Select an appropriate font size
- Use a uniform font per slide
- Have an appropriate number of text lines and points to be made

---

Always use the spell checker

There is nothing worse than slides with incorrect spelling. It gives the impression that you have not really taken the time to prepare the presentation and have simply thrown up anything in front of your audience.

Slide background

A wide range of backgrounds is available as standard in PowerPoint and an infinite number can be constructed with various colours, shades, and textures. As with the layout of text on the slide, it is important to select a combination which enhances and clarifies your presentation. White or yellow text on a blue background is a safe option while red and green may be lost to someone with colour blindness. Figure 5.1 illustrates the problem of using white text on a light textured background – the message is lost completely.

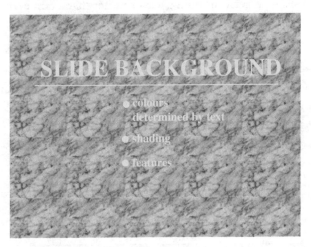

Figure 5.1 Illustration of the problem of using white text on a light textured background.

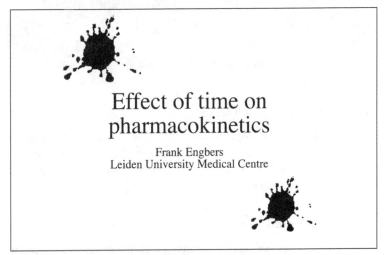

Figure 5.2 Personalised master slide.

Some expert presenters go to considerable lengths to personalise their PowerPoint backgrounds as illustrated in Figure 5.2, which is reputed to have taken several days to get the ink blot shapes exactly correct.

We now get to those features which separate out PowerPoint from other presentation media. These can be used to retain the attention of an audience, but the main danger is that they can also be used to entertain the audience to the extent that they are watching for the next slide transition, or spectacular form of building text, rather than concentrating on the wisdom contained within the slides.

Slide transition

Slides can glide down from above, each side, or below; they can split out, in, and down plus very many other types of transition. It is important to restrict the use of these transitions to avoid providing too much entertainment with the medium rather than education with the content.

Building text

A similar danger lies in the excessive use of different types of text build. These features allow text to be built up in many different ways. Lines of text can be constructed by wiping to the right or left or by dropping in single letters of each word. Text can be flown in from the side, top, or bottom of the slide; spiral effects spin the text out from the centre.

It is important not to overdo the special effects

Save the special effects for the occasions when you want to make an especially important series of points rather than using them indiscriminately throughout your presentation.

Graphics

It is possible to use the graphics functions in PowerPoint to produce simple illustrations such as block and line drawings (Figure 5.3), or to import data from a spreadsheet which can then produce a line graph that can be superimposed on to a block diagram (Figure 5.4).

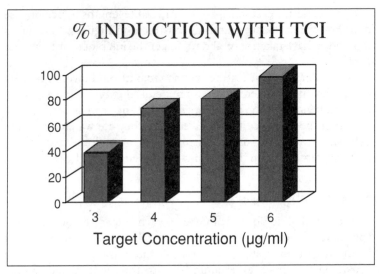

Figure 5.3 The graphic functions in PowerPoint allows simple illustrations to be produced.

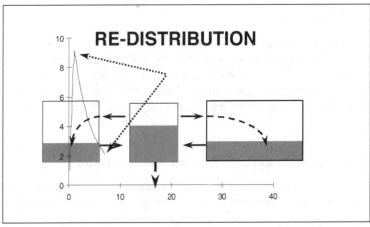

Figure 5.4 Imported data from a spreadsheet is used to produce a line graph which can be superimposed on to a block diagram.

Digital photographs

One of the most useful features of PowerPoint is the ability to insert different components into your presentation. Digital photographs or scanned 35 mm slides can now be projected using XGA resolution and provide excellent quality. Your old 35 mm slide collection of apparatus, patients or pathology can therefore be scanned and stored permanently on a CD-ROM. An image of this type can be inserted on to a slide and then annotated to point out specific points in the illustration (Figure 5.5). Where you do not have scanned images and must use 35 mm slides, the best technique is to stop with a completely black slide in your PowerPoint presentation where you wish to show your 35 mm slides. Then advance your 35 mm slides to show the number you require, finish with a blank 35 mm slide, and continue with your PowerPoint presentation.

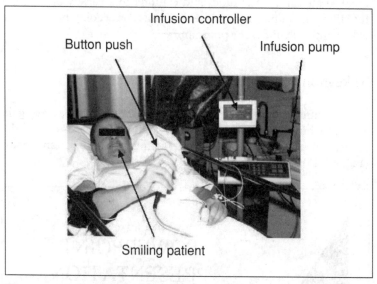

Figure 5.5 Slides can be scanned into PowerPoint and captions added to illustrate each point.

Digital videos

In a similar way to digital photographs, digital video clips can be incorporated into a PowerPoint slide. This is an extremely powerful tool which can be used to illustrate the data in real life by showing a patient having surgery, waking up, or whatever point you wish to demonstrate. The main difficulty with incorporating video and photographic material into your presentation is that the memory requirements increase dramatically. A presentation with seven or eight high-resolution digital photographs and a few video clips may exceed 30 or 40 megabytes in file size.

Run another programme

You may wish to run another programme in the middle of your PowerPoint presentation. This could be a spreadsheet or a special pharmacokinetic simulation programme. Action buttons can be incorporated into your slides and can link to a variety of different functions, including running a different PowerPoint presentation or a completely different programme.

Take-home messages

Use different formats for your slide backgrounds to gain attention but not to entertain your audience. For example, the occasional use of an arrow can highlight an important point (Figure 5.6).

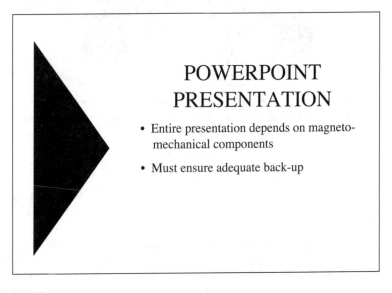

Figure 5.6 Occasional use of a different slide format can be used to highlight a particular point.

Controlling the presentation

The really bad way to start your PowerPoint presentation is to move to the lectern, switch on your laptop and wait while everything starts up, select your presentation file, and then begin. It is much more professional to have your laptop switched on and connected to the PC projector. Have your presentation running but put a completely black slide on first. This will appear as a blank screen to the audience. Advance to the next slide and your show commences. Similarly, it is a poor ending to simply reach the last slide and for your presentation to end with all your slides shown in slide sorter mode. It is better to place another black slide so that when you are finished, again there is a blank screen. Put two black slides in, in case you inadvertently double advance the slide.

The alternative is to press the "B" key on the keyboard which will blank off the screen and the presentation. Pressing once more will restore the screen display. Pressing the "W" key, gives a blank white screen. Forward and backward movement of the slides can be controlled by using the arrow keys. Pressing the "N" key or the spacebar will also advance to the next slide.

Sometimes, the computer is too far from the lectern for you to physically touch the keyboard. This can be solved by using either an infra-red or radio remote control. The receiver may be connected directly to the computer or via the PC projector. Such a system is especially useful when you are using a radio tie microphone since you can then move freely about the stage and also use the remote mouse to move the arrow around your slide to point out different features.

Jumping to conclusions

It is extremely important that you have the courtesy to keep to your allotted time. But few of us have such perfect timing. PowerPoint can help you to produce perfectly timed presentations. Use a timer to warn of two to three minutes left and know the slide number of your conclusion slide. When your timer warns that you have just the correct time to present your conclusions, enter the slide number of your conclusion slide and press the <return> key. You will immediately skip any other slides and go directly to the slide number that you entered.

This method requires you to know the number of the conclusion slide at the start of your presentation. A better way is to use an action button on your master slide. This can be a small semi-transparent area which will only really be visible to you. It is set up in the Action settings to hyperlink to the slide in your presentation labelled "conclusions". When you are presenting, all your slides will have this small action button and when you move your mouse pointer over the button, and press the right button, the system will automatically jump to your "conclusions" slide, no matter how many other slides are in between.

And finally

You should have a check list to go through before you give your presentation which will ensure that everything is in place (see Box 5.3).

Box 5.3 Final preparations

- Arrive at the auditorium early

- Check the projector interfaces correctly to your system

- Check the mains power is connected to your system

- Set up the presentation with a black slide as the first, or press the "B" key to give a blank screen

- Relax – you are ready to give a superb presentation

There is only one way to become familiar with this type of presentation and that is to practice again and again. Observe what others do in their presentations and then ask how they managed to do it. It must be obvious that PowerPoint is unique in providing a phenomenally wide range of possibilities to produce a complete disaster of a presentation. However, it is a powerful communication tool which offers, at present, the ultimate to dazzle, astonish, and to hold the attention of your audience. If you cannot hold their attention, then your presentation will not make the points you wish to your audience. A further advantage is that the slides in a PowerPoint presentation are *always* the correct way round.

Summary

- Ensure that you have back-up material in case your PowerPoint presentation crashes

- Use a standard presentation template to avoid producing confusing slides

- Set up the computer equipment before beginning your presentation

- Use the timer on PowerPoint to warn you when your presentation time is coming to an end

6 How to appear on stage

ALAN MARYON DAVIS

So you have worked hard on your presentation. You've honed it down to the key points. You've sorted out a few jokes. You've got great graphics. And you've timed it to a tee. In short, you've done about as much with it as you can, and as talks go, it is not at all bad.

But what about you yourself? How will you come across? Many a potentially excellent talk has been scuppered by inept presenting. We've all had to endure speakers who can't be heard, or who look all wrong, or who display some thoroughly irritating mannerism that completely distracts from what they're trying to get across.

How can you avoid such pitfalls? Better still, how can you appear slick, confident and impressive on stage? Or, perhaps more realistically, how can you at least make sure that you don't get too much in the way of your own presentation?

Here are a few basic tips – most of which I have to confess I learnt the hard way – to help you avoid the likeliest own-goals.

Get there early

The first piece of advice is: make sure you arrive in plenty of time. We've all seen the consequences of turning up at the last minute. The chairman looks anxiously at the clock, wondering whether to bring the coffee break forward. Kerfuffle at the back of the hall. Speaker bursts in, scattering notes and overheads. Stumbles onto stage, knocks over microphone, scrabbles for projector switch, shoves on first overhead upside-down, and generally kyboshes the entire proceedings.

You can avoid all that by getting there early. There are several advantages:

- It gives you an opportunity to pick up the "mood" of the meeting and the issues that may have a bearing on your talk.

- It demonstrates to the gathering that you have more than just a passing commitment to the subject.
- It allows you time to familiarise yourself with the stage set-up, podium, panel table, microphones, and projection gear.
- It focuses your mind on the task ahead.
- It helps to calm your nerves and those of the organisers.

Sounds OK?

Grappling with an unfamiliar sound system is a classic elephant trap for hapless speakers. The usual disasters are failing to switch on the microphone, failing to make sure that it's pointing in the right direction, constantly clunking the lead, or speaking so closely that you sound like a Dalek with laryngitis in a thunderstorm.

Spend a few minutes before your session starts to do a sound check – and if necessary make a few adjustments. If you're using a microphone on a stand– either a floor-stand, table-stand or fixed to the podium – adjust it so that it's pointing at your mouth, but is positioned slightly to one side of the direct line of fire of your breath as you speak. This is to avoid "popping" – those periodic explosions accompanying every "P" that punctuates a presentation. The microphone should be about 6 in (15 cm) from your mouth, and on the side nearer the screen because if you happen to turn your head away from it, to look at the screen for example, your voice may disappear. To check the set-up, say a few words. Instead of the time-worn "testing, one, two, three, testing", I would recommend "Peter Piper picked a peck of pickled pepper" to sort out the pops from the snaps and crackles.

The lapel microphone may be a marvel of miniaturisation, but it can cause tons of trouble. First, there's the agony of where to clip it – a particular challenge for presenters without lapels. Women often find themselves in this awkward situation – and occasionally have to resort to holding the thing in position. With a radio microphone, the box of works can provide an even more difficult problem. If you have no pocket handy, you should be able to rest it on the podium. But if there is no podium, or if you're standing at the overhead projector, you could find yourself with both hands full. I remember one particular female presenter who performed a remarkably nimble impromptu juggling act with a clip-on microphone, its black box, and a profusion of wildly haphazard overheads. And then there is the pitfall of failing to disconnect yourself at the end of your talk. This can either result in half your apparel being yanked away as you attempt to leave the podium, or, with a radio mike, the much more disastrous consequence of inadvertently leaving the thing switched on and accidentally telling everyone what dumb questions you felt you'd just been asked.

Looking good

Half the battle with successful presenting is to look good. By that I don't mean you have to don your best Armani – which might provoke antibodies in some quarters. I mean looking self-assured and confident, knowing how to stand and move, and generally having poise and style. If you appear to be comfortably in command of the situation it will help people focus more on what you have to say rather than the struggle you're having saying it.

As far as dress is concerned, this clearly depends on the type of meeting. What would be appropriate for a small informal lunchtime session for GPs might not be at all right for an international conference. My advice is to try to strike a balance between what you perceive is expected by the organisers, and what you feel comfortable in. If there is a golden rule, I would say it's not to wear anything that either distracts or detracts from the message or impression you want to put across. So, fight temptation and leave that favourite ultra-loud tie or those knock-'em-dead sparklers firmly at home.

Standing and moving

It was once rather unfairly observed of the accident-prone US ex-President Gerald Ford that he couldn't walk down stairs and chew gum at the same time. Certainly many speakers do develop acute dystaxia when they get up on stage and have to cope with talking, following their notes, pressing buttons, changing overheads and pointing at things on the screen, all more-or-less simultaneously.

Good preparation and rehearsal can prevent most difficulties in this respect. I've already mentioned being familiar with the set-up, so that you know exactly which buttons to press. It also pays to have your notes (if you have any) clearly page-numbered, with bold headings, so that you can quickly navigate your way through them and instantly find your place again when you look up at your audience. They should also have clear prompts to cue each slide. Overheads should have their backing sheets already removed (to avoid them looking too freshly made), and be interleaved with plain paper (so you can see what they are, and also to prevent them sticking together). They should be numbered (just in case you drop the lot) and, if possible, already placed in position on the OHP projector side-table, with a space to stack them again after use.

As soon as you hear yourself being introduced, go straight into successful presenter mode and walk confidently up those steps, smiling at the chairman who hopefully has said a few nice things about you. When you reach your position, place your notes, check the microphone, smile at the audience, and launch forth.

If you're using slides or computer graphics, the chances are you'll be speaking from the podium. Most speakers find the podium quite a comfort. Not only does it conveniently hold your notes, but it also gives you something to lean on in a casual, relaxed fashion, emanating calm professionalism. And it's a shield that you can literally and metaphorically hide behind, so that you don't feel so exposed.

But others regard the podium as a millstone, encumbering their performance. They much prefer the freedom to move about, made possible either by a radio microphone or a very loud voice. This provides a wonderful opportunity to be more expressive, engaging and even dramatic. But be careful not to over-egg the cake. If you do too much strutting and fretting, it can divert attention from what you're trying to communicate.

If you've got lots of overheads, you'll obviously be spending most of the time at the projector. You should either be wearing a lapel microphone or have a standing microphone placed there for you – otherwise you'll be constantly darting back and forth to the podium.

There are several points to watch with presenting overheads:

- Glance at the screen when you place the first one, to make sure that it's properly positioned. Tilting, out-of-frame or back-to-front overheads are irritating.
- After that, try not to look at the screen again. Because you're right in front of it, you'll be turning your back on the audience, which doesn't look good.
- If you need to point to something, use a pen or pencil to indicate it directly on the overhead itself rather than pointing at the screen image.

- Place the pointer in position and leave it there. Don't wave it about – again, that's irritating.
- And as we've said elsewhere, each overhead should have no more than about five brief bullet points in a large font size.

When wielding a laser pointer, usually with 35 mm slides, don't make the classic mistake of holding it at arm's length as though it is about to go off. This almost guarantees wild fluctuations. Keep it close to you, preferably braced against your trunk to steady it. And avoid a surfeit of artistry in the form of wild loops and swirls.

How to speak

The key points are:

- Be audible. If you can't be heard, your words are wasted.
- Be intelligible. If your words can't be understood, the audience is wasted.
- Be engaging. If you don't hold the audience's attention, your slot in the programme is wasted.

So don't mumble. Don't speak in a monotone. Keep your chin up, and project your voice to the back of the room.

Preferably use brief notes or your slides as a prompt rather than reading word-for-word from a full text. Leave plenty of pauses, especially after making a key point. It gives the audience a chance to take things in properly, and you a chance to catch your breath.

Sound and look enthusiastic, or at least interested in your own talk. Nothing turns off an audience more swiftly than a speaker who emanates utter boredom and would clearly rather be somewhere else. If *you* don't look as though you believe in what you're saying, nobody else will.

On the other hand, don't swing too far in the other direction. Stressing every other word can be very wearing, a sing-song inflection can be thoroughly irritating, and an over-indulgence in arm-waving an exercise in distraction. So, plenty of enthusiasm, commitment, passion even – but not at the cost of losing the message. Ranting and raving is all very well, but only in moderation.

Eye contact

It is important to get the eye contact right from the outset – it makes a big difference to how well you engage your audience. Here are a few tips:

- Don't just talk to your notes or the screen.
- Don't stare at the floor, ceiling, clock, or out of the window.
- Don't just address the front row or two. The rest of the audience will feel excluded.
- Don't fix your gaze too much on someone who seems to be paying attention. You may lose the only friend you have.
- Do engage with all parts of the auditorium – middle, front, back, left and right – so that you draw the whole audience into your circle of confidence.

And finally ... a word about coping with nerves

You may have done all the right things – carefully prepared your talk, rehearsed a few times in front of your colleagues, arrived at the venue early, checked all the systems – and still find that you're a bag of nerves as you wait to be called up on stage. What can you do to restore inner calm?

I wish I knew. I still have this problem to some extent after goodness knows how many appearances on stage, both in my capacity as a doctor and as a member of the humorous singing group Instant Sunshine – despite the fact that with the latter I'm meant to appear a bit haphazard because it's part of the act. Indeed, I'm so apprehensive about public speaking that I even put off getting married for several years simply because I couldn't face having to make a speech to thank the bridesmaids.

So I'm hardly the person to advise on this. Of course, I could simply rattle off the usual list of relaxation tips – you know – all the stuff about deep breathing, imagining waves lapping on the shore, tensing and relaxing your muscles, reciting a silent mantra. But you're probably as unconvinced about all that as I am.

My advice is to just do it. Throw yourself into it. Ride the tiger. Harness the adrenalin to give your talk that vital bit of edge. The chances are you won't be looking anything like as nervous as you feel. And notwithstanding what I've just said, there is light at the end of the tunnel. It actually does get easier with practice.

Summary

- Make sure you arrive in plenty of time
- Spend time before your presentation to do a sound check
- Look self-assured
- When speaking be audible, intelligible and engaging
- Maintain eye contact with the audience

7 How to sell a message

MARTIN GODFREY

Having a message and then selling it are central to the process of getting your point across – surely the main aim of any presentation. This chapter will help you to identify your messages, create them succinctly, and get them across effectively.

Unfortunately the word "message", used in the context of a meeting, doesn't usually do much for the average medic. It conjures up a variety of unappealing mental pictures, ranging from the archetypal Armani-suited marketing man spinning a story for some corporate seminar, to the American evangelist proselytising to a football stadium of believers. Surely medics don't have messages; they have ideas or facts or data or something much less commercial.

But I can reassure you: messages are OK. Messages are what you need to communicate effectively. In fact, no successful speaker or factual writer has ever gone very far without consciously or unconsciously being very good at creating messages and selling them. All the best politicians, journalists, business leaders, professors, dictators, etc, sell messages as a central part of what they know they have to do.

So let's start with the message. Before you do anything else in preparing for your presentation you must be clear about your messages. Use them to create a skeleton on which the rest can hang.

What is a message? A message is a simple statement of the main thing or things you want to say. It is, in effect, a succinct summary of the point you are making.

At their best, messages become virtual slogans: "Vote Conservative" or "Ken Livingstone for Mayor". But they can be longer and do not necessarily have to appear as such in your presentation – they are merely what you would want to be left with if the whole thing was distilled down to a complete minimum.

So a message might be: "The Conservative party stands for law and order" or "Ken Livingstone will not nationalise the Underground". Try not to overcomplicate.

Journalists are trained to try to put their main messages into the "introduction" – the first paragraph – of their news article. Since they have to make sense grammatically, these introductions tend to be a little longer than the raw message. But the process of arriving at the gist of what they want to say can be used by anyone trying to cut through large amounts of verbiage to reach the key point underneath.

One useful tip to do this is to imagine you are walking down the street and you see your mother just getting on to a bus. You have something important to tell her, but the bus is moving off and thus you have only seconds to summarise what you want to say as you run breathlessly behind her. It's that sound-bite, that "in a nutshell sentence", that will give you your main message should you be uncertain of its real nature.

How many messages? As a general rule, it is best not to have too many messages in a presentation. People can easily get lost if you are trying to say too much. The old adage "keep it simple, stupid" is a good one to remember.

So, have one, or at the most, two or three key messages – never more. If you feel you need to use more, you will probably find that many of the others are merely subsidiary to those initial key messages and can be developed as supporting points. If you still have more, then make two presentations.

Now you have your key messages, how are you going to sell them? First, you have to really understand your audience. Put yourself in their shoes and ask yourself the following questions as if you were being presented to by yourself:

- How will your ideas help me?
- What are the facts and where are the snags?
- Do I agree or disagree?
- What are my needs?

One of the great insights about effective presenting is that if you are really going to sell to your audience they must connect with the benefits of what you are selling. So you must understand their individual needs and tailor your message-sell accordingly.

For example, if you are selling a Porsche you should understand that the needs of most of those buying it will revolve around getting from London to Manchester as fast and with as much excitement as possible. They are not that interested in whether the car has side impact safety features or a three-year warranty.

So, your message is that the Porsche you are selling is the fastest and most exciting car on the road. Selling it as the safest car on the road might equally be true, but it isn't what they want to hear – it's not what they *need*. Understand your audience's needs and address them directly.

Let's go back to the Conservatives. You are selling the message that the Conservative party is the party of law and order and you are presenting to a group of policemen. What they need is to have a party that will support them in doing their job. What they want is more policemen, better pay, and a judiciary that has the power to convict.

But what if the audience is made up entirely of medical students? They might simply want more policemen on the beat, more neighbourhood watch schemes, and similar things.

But you can just imagine how difficult it might be to sell such a message to a group of students. They are suspicious, and law and order is not necessarily something that medical school students really think should be increased. They will more than likely be suspicious and only vaguely in touch with their own needs in this area. That's where the next trick to effective message-selling comes in. Don't sell *features*, sell *benefits*.

More policemen is a feature; fewer manpower shortages and thus less stress is the benefit to the policeman or woman.

More beat policemen is a feature; more manpower to prevent burglaries around the halls of residence is a benefit.

A 4-litre engine is a feature; 0–60 in 3·5 seconds is a benefit.

In other words, people buy solutions not things or services. A man who goes into a DIY store looking for a 1·5 cm diameter drill bit may not know it, but in reality what he is buying is a 1·5 cm hole.

So, we have clear, simple messages, an understanding of the audience's needs, and a desire to sell benefits, not features. How do you put all that together into a winning presentation?

No two presentations are the same, but there are some basics that you should attempt to ensure are covered.

- Introduce the presentation – highlight your key message(s) and ensure your audience is left with a clear idea of how you are going to address the topic. A map of your presentation is very useful here. Return to it frequently so your audience doesn't lose its way and get bored.

- Follow a presentation process. The classic method is to first analyse where you are, discuss where you want to be, outline the options and then deliver your chosen solution.
- Don't have too much verbiage on the slides. Your slides are effectively just wallpaper allowing you to highlight certain key points. Never have more than three words per bullet point and try to include lots of pictures.
- Make sure the benefits you are highlighting are clearly shown.
- Always summarise (in fact it is a good idea to summarise regularly throughout the presentation) and ensure your key messages are all in there.
- Ask your audience directly if they got the message. If you discover they haven't understood, let alone bought, the message then at least you have one last chance to get things right.

Lastly, a few words on presentation style. A great presentation can be lost if the presenter is not interacting with the audience, while a poor presentation can become a great one with an engaged audience.

Actors are often taught that to really interact with an audience they need to demonstrate a level of emotion and animation. To help analyse this emotional element, a ladder of seven emotional presentation styles was developed by a French actor in the 1960s:

Level one: *Total exhaustion.*

Level two: *The Californian.* Very relaxed, very friendly, but to the point. This style puts your audience at their ease and allows you to appear confident and unthreatening.

Level three: *The stage manager.* This alludes to the neutral figures in black outfits who walk briskly onto the stage, move a piece of furniture then walk off again. They show neutral emotion. This is the state in which most people present and not surprisingly they do not succeed in connecting with their audience. Typically the presenter speaks in a monotone with an unemotional voice with few movements of any kind.

Level four: *The director.* Animated, direct and sure footed. Probably the ideal presentation style. The presenter feels as if he or she is in command of the room, looking at each member of the audience as he/she makes a point and only moving eye contact once the point has been made.

Level five: *There may be a bomb in the room.* Very high energy, but usually too much for a normal presentation.

Level six: *We found the bomb*. High, negative energy levels.
Level seven: *The nervous breakdown*.

Always try to be in either the Californian or the director mode –
years of practice has shown that these styles work. And don't forget
to be positive and interested, ensuring that there is plenty of
inflection in your voice. When you get to your key messages, try
pausing to heighten the level of interest; emphasise them and, if
necessary, repeat them to ensure you get the point across. And
remember to really feel interested in what you are saying. This may
sound fundamental, but it is amazing how dislocated many of us
become when we are having to present. If you aren't showing
interest, it's certain none of your audience will be!

In summary, then, successfully selling messages in a presentation
involves the development of a very few simple messages;
understanding the audience's needs; selling benefits, not features,
and ensuring (through practice) the correct projection of emotion
and interest.

Summary

- Be clear about what your messages are and try to keep
  them simple
- Only have two or three key messages in your presentation
- Ensure that the audience understands the benefits of the
  messages
- Maintain the right projection of emotion and interest

Further reading

Fisher R, Ury W, Patton B. *Getting to yes*. Century Business Books, 1991
Kelcher M. *Better communication skills for work*. BBC Books, 1992.
Senge P M . *The fifth discipline: the art and practice of the learning organisation*.
Century Business Books, 1990

8 How to deal with questions

SIR ALEXANDER MACARA

"We are in danger to be called to question"
Acts of the Apostles, xix, 40

It is to be hoped that readers will find that questions provide opportunities rather than dangers.

Like ancient Gaul, this chapter falls into three parts: how to answer questions after giving a presentation at a meeting; how to handle interviews from the "media"; and how to cope with a "brains trust" or panel discussion.

Questions following a presentation

The story is told of an eminent physicist who had reluctantly accepted an invitation to address a predictably tiresome meeting. He was driven there by his favourite postgraduate student. On arrival, his disinclination to speak overcame any sense of obligation, and he decided to rest in his car whilst sending the student, armed with his PowerPoint presentation, to give the lecture. The eager acolyte coped competently with the presentation itself and with agreeably animated discussion until he was fazed by a particularly difficult challenge. "The question is of rather too general a nature to require my expertise", he replied, "but I will invite my chauffeur to deal with it."

The credibility of the story aside, it does raise some salutary points. Obviously, one should try to avoid accepting unwelcome invitations and, if one has to delegate the invitation to a colleague, albeit armed with your prepared script, bear in mind that he might have problems dealing with questions. Moreover, care must be taken not to underestimate the intelligence or knowledge of the audience; invariably someone will know more about some aspects of the subject than the speaker.

So, to our task. How should one approach audience's questions after a presentation?

- Prepare as for the presentation itself by seeking to master the subject. You can choose what to say or not to say in the presentation, but you can only speculate about questions, and "being called in question" clearly presents more dangers than the presentation itself. Invited to address French professors of social medicine in the elegant Chateau de Longchamps in Paris about a European Association to which I wanted to recruit them, I was unexpectedly bidden to speak in French. All went well enough until questions came – more fast than thick. The chairman came to the rescue: "They all speak English, *mon ami*, so it is only fair now to switch to your language." The problem is, however, more often with the question itself than with the language in which it is couched, so one's preparation should not only cover the immediate ground of the subject but survey the hinterland. For example, if addressing "clinical advances in late onset diabetes", one should review the epidemiology, the history of the diagnosis, treatment and management of the disease, together with its effect on the person as a whole, its relationship to other conditions, and its social, occupational, and economic implications.
- Conduct a reconnaissance of the expected audience before preparing.
- Speculate about questions. Rehearse what you might choose to say in reply.
- On the day, dress up rather than down. Beverley Baxter once observed that "by your dress you show respect". Turning up in a dinner jacket and finding everyone else in casual smart attire, the late Sir John Brotherston – then CMO Scotland – explained, "I have just come from the office". Conversely, failing to wear a dinner jacket to a "black tie dinner" is not so easily explained away. A jacket and tie can always be removed if appropriate; indeed, it may be effective after a formal presentation to slip off one's jacket before knuckling down to questions.
- Ascertain whether reporters are to be present and, if so, whom they represent. At a typically sparsely attended AGM which I was waiting to address, it was agreed that those attending should constitute the executive committee *en bloc*. The scrupulous secretary insisted on listing the names, thereby

identifying an unknown young person as being from the medical newspaper, *PULSE.*

- Make your mark with the chairman: if a woman, ascertain whether she wishes to be addressed traditionally as "Madam Chairman" or, as in contemporary parlance, as an inanimate object with four legs. The chairman has the power to make or break the occasion – and the speaker. If in doubt about any of the arrangements, seek the chairman's advice.
- Seek to give an impression of modest self-confidence; be positive, not negative. Allow an element of self-deprecation. Irony is acceptable, sarcasm is not.
- Speak simply, with appropriate colloquial language but not slang. Practise conciseness and clarity as distinct from brevity and over-simplification. Fluency is admirable but a stammer, which can suddenly afflict anyone in a difficult situation, can be turned to good account. The distinguished and much loved paediatrician, Freddie Miller, who had a particularly engaging stammer, used to relieve his hearers of any embarrassment by claiming that it was an advantage – "it gives one time to think".
- Indulge in spontaneous humour if you have the gift. Guard against giving gratuitous offence by insensitivity about age, gender, religion, or race.
- Above all, try to keep calm under stress, however provoked you may be. A soft answer can turn away wrath and, more importantly, does nothing to diminish one's authority. Try to obtain, and maintain, eye contact with the audience throughout. Heaven defend one from the high platform, the scattered remote audience, the dim lighting, except, infuriatingly, in front of one's own eyes. In such a situation – sadly increasingly common – one can only do one's best. Ignore the spoiler who is muttering disapprovingly and speak directly to the empathetic listener.
- When the question is put, listen to it but try also to assess why it is asked; body language will often give a clue. Does the questioner genuinely want information or is he or she trying to impress? Be sensitive to the effect of your answer on the audience as a whole; including any reporters. In any event, answer the question which is asked (you are not a politician).
- Correct any mistaken assumptions in the question.
- The chairman may summarise, or seek to clarify, the question; beware any change in its meaning or purpose, in which case your reply will call for diplomacy.

- Do not launch into a second presentation; leave people wanting more. Allow room for a supplementary question.
- If you consider the question stupid, be courteous and explain the relevant facts as though it had been sensible.
- If the question is too profound, you may have to regret that lack of time (has anyone ordered breakfast?) precludes a reply in depth. If the question is very wide, lack of time similarly precludes a reply in breadth.
- If the questioner is disconcertingly knowledgeable, you may invite his or her own opinion/explanation/information.
- What if one does not know the answer to the question? The celebrated Scots dramatist, James Bridie, a "chronic" medical student in those halcyon days when universities were relaxed about examinations, when asked the external relations of the knee joint, replied, "I do not know the external relations of the knee joint, but the external relations of the elbow joint are . . . ". Not a bad try, but better to be honest and admit that you do not know. Ask if someone else can help – perhaps the questioner?

How should you handle the individual who interrupts your presentation? You may have been forewarned about the bearded chap in a red shirt and green tie, and are therefore prepared. The chairman may come to the rescue but only you can decide whether or not to give way. Do either with good grace. An effective ploy is to claim that you are coming to that particular point later, whether or not you have any such intention.

On being interviewed

Keith Joseph was a disconcertingly honest intellectual, best remembered for his reorganisation of the NHS as Secretary of State in the Health Administration in the early 1970s. The story is told of his first television interview in the early days of that revealing medium, when he was a new junior minister. He answered every question unguardedly, and had the insight at the end to observe that the interview had been disastrous. "Yes, Sir Keith", replied his interviewer, "I am afraid it was." "Then we must do it again". "But, Sir Keith, it was *live*". "That is why I want do it again".

Today's politicians are trained to deal with interviews, especially on television. Keith Joseph's experience reminds us of the crucial importance of knowing whether the interview is being recorded or broadcast "live", or whether there may be an opportunity to see or hear it in advance and to make changes. As with questions from any audience, one needs to know who one's readers, listeners, or viewers are likely to be, whom the interviewer is representing, and what the objective of the interview is. It is wise to assume that interviewers are knowledgeable and that they may be hoping to present a preconceived angle. One also needs to know whether any colleagues – or others, especially if potential adversaries – are to be appearing alongside you and, if so, what contribution they are likely to make, and what is to be the order of appearance. Prepare a number of points – five at most. However you may be provoked, try to remain studiously courteous, but cautious: exceptions prove the rule. Remember that it is *your* subject (or you should not be there), and *your* interview. The honour of your specialty, your practice, hospital, or university, may be in your hands.

Your *aide memoire* should include the following additional points.

- Make your remarks appropriate to the audience, whether professional or general. Avoid jargon except for a specially knowledgeable audience.
- Correct any mistakes by the interviewer unless the matter is trivial and correction would be petty.
- Beware of pitfalls, for example, "So what you are saying is..." when it is not, or the multiple point question which is unanswerable in limited time; reply, "The main point(s) is (are)...".
- Take care with statistics: they should be told only when they are telling and if in doubt, leave them out. Keep them simple, for example, "half" rather than "approximately 50% give or take a point or two".
- Do not say, "I have *x* points" (although you do). You will look foolish when you fall short of the expected number.
- Never denigrate a rival or opponent.

The newspaper or journal interview

There are two specific related points.

- Avoid talking "off the record" or "unattributably" even when invited to do so, unless you are very confident that the reporter is someone you can trust to resist the temptation to pull off a

scoop on the strength of your indiscretion.
- Assume that anything you say may be quoted.

The radio or television interview

Whichever the medium, try to ascertain how much time you will have. The duration of the interview may depend upon how cogent and convincing you are in reply to the first question. Television can be particularly brutal in cutting you off in mid-sentence either on the spot or in the cutting room. You may have to persuade the interviewer that you have something to say in order to secure the interview at all. The onus may be on you to secure a favourable interview. When Fergus Walsh, the veteran television interviewer, was reporting the profession's Core Values Conference in 1994, he was clearly sceptical as to whether we had anything "new" to say. One was able to represent that, for the first time, the medical profession had explicitly acknowledged its responsibility, not only to individual patients and to the honour of the profession, but to society as a whole, which led to the desired discussion about scarcity of resources and rationing.

There are rules, or at least tips, which are particularly relevant to radio and television.

- Say less rather than more; an arresting short reply to the opening question will invite further questions and secure more time to get your points across within the pre-set limit.
- Be prepared to back up your assertions or claims crisply with evidence or examples. Taking refuge in reassertion or waffle will leave you sounding or looking very foolish.
- Do not say, "Speaking personally, I myself think...". Tautology apart, "I think" suggests you do not *know*. Do not start with "well", or use fillers such as "um..., er..., em..". Avoid "you know" like the plague; they do not, you are supposed to be telling them.
- Sound (and, on television, look) convincing and enthusiastic.
- Be pleasant to the interviewer whatever your true feelings, he (or she) can make you sound better or worse than you deserve.
- When you have finished, stop.

Each medium has its advantages and disadvantages. Hence, general rules apply to both, but there are specific points to bear in mind for each. Radio is less subject to distraction – for everyone concerned – than television. Radio puts a premium on the voice and television on the image. Vision can either distract from the message or enhance it. One's style of dress and address reinforce each other. Competent professionalism is the passport to success. Ignore the camera and look at the interviewer, who is usually more interesting; moreover, you need to read his or her body language. Do not fall for the pregnant pause and feel you have to fill a gap with some ill-considered irrelevance. Take care with your physical presentation. Stand full square with feet firmly on the ground, or sit upright in your chairman, not rocking it or yourself. Acknowledge your introduction and dismissal with a smile. You may be shown going about your business to set the scene for the interview. Appear brisk and business-like. It helps to carry an impressive-looking folder, but not a pile of books which suggests that you cannot cope without a mobile library. Avoid steps.

The brains trust or panel

The eminent philosopher Professor Joad, a resident member of the original pre-television era BBC Brains Trust, once famously recast the question "What is life?" as: "What *is* life?" The point of this anecdote is that a panel discussion is a different genre from the one-to-one question and answer session or interview. It often offers the opportunity to turn a question round in such a way as to give a more stimulating and useful answer than the original question permits. However, your answer should be no less relevant to the original question, and should not be calculated to score over the other members of the panel, although it may have that effect. No matter, there is an inevitable element of rivalry – not always friendly – between the members of a panel, all of whom are anxious to reveal their knowledge or conceal their ignorance. "The question is, which is to be master?" to quote Humpty Dumpty.

The challenge is to strike the right note. It is death to discussion for everyone to sing in unison, but discordant clashes can be equally destructive. Panel members should resist the temptation to interrupt their colleagues, however provoked, but should be prepared to respond when invited to help them out. Wit or originality always enhances proceedings, as does a telling anecdote. As in other situations the chairman, however self-effacing, is the key figure, particularly in controlling anyone seeking to dominate proceedings and in encouraging less assertive participants. The chairman will usually decide upon the order of batting and move quickly to another member of the panel when one is stumped.

Sometimes the chairman will throw the question open, and an instant decision is required. Do you jump in, or wait? If you know the answer, have a go while the others are thinking; they will have to follow your lead or justify doing otherwise. If you do not have anything to say, save your breath in the hope that others will give you a clue, or an opportunity to agree with them – the sincerest form of flattery – adding that you have nothing to add, which will please everyone, including the person waiting with contrived patience to pose the next question.

Let the last word be with Sir Toby Belch: "I can say little more than I have studied".

Summary

- When preparing a presentation, prepare for the types of questions that might be asked afterwards

- Make sure you cater for the particular audience you are addressing

- When being interviewed prepare up to five points and try to remain courteous but cautious

- If you are a member of a panel respond with a relevant answer and do not interrupt your colleagues

Further reading

Media Tips. *BMA Public Affairs Division*, 2000.

9 How not to give a presentation

RICHARD SMITH

The invitation arrives. You are invited to speak on the same programme as the Pope, Bill Clinton, Madonna, and Chomsky. Beside yourself with excitement, you forget that you've had these sort of invitations before and that for some strange reason none of the famous people ever turn up. They are all replaced by people you've never heard of who turn out to be even more boring than you. Having accepted the invitation, you get your own back by forgetting it completely. Two years later – 15 minutes before you are due to start speaking in Florence – you receive a phone call at your office in London asking where you are.

"I'm sorry," you answer lamely, "I forgot."

"Don't worry," answers the cheery voice at the end, "We'll just ask Madonna to speak for 20 minutes longer. The audience of millionaire surgeons will be disappointed you're not here, but extra Madonna will be some compensation."

Far from ruining this presentation, you may have improved the surgeons' conference. But forgetting altogether that you agreed to speak is a good way to make a mess of your presentation. A variant is to arrive late. Don't arrive too late because they will simply have cancelled your session, probably sending a thrill of pleasure through an audience facing the prospect of five consecutive speakers. The best thing is to arrive about eight minutes late when the chairman has exhausted his puny supply of jokes and is just starting to introduce the next speaker. Rush up to the podium, waving your hands furiously, and apologise profusely. If you can, trip over on the way. Once at the podium you can either spend five minutes searching for your notes or else say: "I'm sorry, I've not had time to give my 87 slides to the man in the projector room." Or you could try saying "I'm sure that my PowerPoint presentation is on this disc somewhere", as you project onto the screen a list of hundreds of similar file names.

My initial point is that there are many, perhaps infinite, ways to give a bad presentation. Tolstoy writes in the first line of Anna Karenina that "All happy families resemble one another, but each unhappy family is unhappy in its own way". The same may be true for presentations. Good ones resemble each other, but bad ones come in many forms.

Preparing for a bad presentation

One way to prepare for a bad presentation is not to prepare at all. Step up to the plate, open your mouth, and see what comes out. With luck your talk will be an incoherent ramble. This is, however, a high risk strategy because spontaneity may catch you out. Most medical presentations are so premeditated that spontaneity may inspire both your audience and you. Inspiration must be avoided at all costs. Similarly you might be caught out by truth. "I've been asked to promote this new drug but actually I'd be fearful of throwing it into the Thames because it might poison the few homunculus fish that survive there." Truth is compelling to an audience, even if mumbled.

A really bad presentation needs careful preparation. A useful standby is to prepare for the wrong audience. If asked to speak to Italians, speak in German. If the audience is made up of 15-year-olds then prepare a complex talk that would baffle a collection of Nobel Prize winners. It's much the best strategy to give an overcomplicated presentation. "Nobody ever lost money underestimating the public's intelligence," said Barnum, Richard Nixon, or somebody, and so you may be surprised by how well your grossly oversimplified presentation is received by your audience of professors.

Be sure to prepare a presentation that is the wrong length. Too long is much the best. Most of the audience will be delighted if your talk is too short, not least because it may provide more opportunity for them to hear their own voices. But something that is too long always works, even if what you are saying is full of wit and wisdom.

Another trick is to ignore the topic you are given. Simply give the bad presentation that you have honed to the point of perfection by giving it time and time again and deleting anything that raises a flicker of interest. With luck most of the audience will have heard it several times before.

Extra help for your bad presentation is to send the organisers in advance a very long and dull CV. Your bad presentation may be given a tremendous boost by the chairman reading out your whole boring life story in a monotone. With luck you might find yourself beginning your presentation after you were supposed to finish. That always depresses an audience.

Aids to a bad presentation

When it comes to aids, standards are rising for those who want to give bad presentations. Indeed, it is probably impossible to give a truly awful presentation without aids. This is an area where new technology is enormously beneficial. First rate bad presentations are usually multimedia: poorly filmed videos that are long and incomprehensible; tapes that are inaudible; music that is out of tune; props that can't be found and then break; and PowerPoint presentations that use every feature the software offers. Satellite links that keep breaking up can often be the icing on the cake of a bad presentation.

Bad slides are the traditional standby of a bad presentation. There must be far too many. They must contain too much information and be too small for even those in the front row to read. Flash them up as fast as you can manage, making sure that they are in the wrong order with some upside down. Include lots of data and complicated graphs, and be sure to say at some point: "I know that this slide breaks all the rules but ... " Ideally there should be little connection between what you are saying and what is on the slide. A good trick, especially with a politically correct audience, is to insert a slide of a naked woman and say something like "My beautiful assistant is, I'm sure you will all agree, a little top heavy." Don't, however, start a riot – otherwise your presentation will be universally agreed to be the best and most memorable.

PowerPoint presentations will usually be preferable to slides because they allow more information to be presented faster, can use a wider range of fonts and colours, and can include moving and flashing signals that can easily be designed to add to the complexity and subtract any meaning that might be getting through.

Unusual aids – such as animals or children – sometimes work. Try introducing all your children plus your pets and parents to the audience. Well done, it might make everybody cringe and create new highs in bad presentations.

Making your bad presentation

The essence of a bad presentation is to be boring. Anything that isn't boring will detract from your bad presentation. Don't wear interesting or unusual clothes. Never look at the audience. Mumble your presentation, and preferably read it. A presentation that is read will usually be satisfyingly bad, but for the full effect you should have long complicated sentences with dozens of subclauses. Try for something as complex as Proust, but get the grammar wrong. Then put all the emphases in the wrong place to ensure that your audience can't understand what you're saying.

Try to torture your audience. Speak for about 10 minutes, and then say: "This is what I'm going to talk about." Then after another 20 minutes say: "I'm now coming to my central point...." Ten minutes later, start saying "Finally". Say it at least five times in the next 15 minutes.

One of the best ways to be boring is to speak for too long. If the chairman tries to stop you, say something like "This is very important". You will, of course, make sure that it isn't important because important things may not be sufficiently boring. It's best to concentrate on the unimportant but to speak with great pomposity. Arrogance and pomposity always enhance a bad presentation. You could also try insulting your audience, but this could be dangerous – because it may become interesting. An electric atmosphere, even if it's electric with anger and embarrassment, is a sure sign that your bad presentation has failed.

Winding down

A truly bad presentation rarely produces any questions. Most people just want to get away. If you do get questions, you may have failed. But all is not lost. By sticking to the basic rules of being boring and overcomplicated and speaking for too long you may be able to rescue your bad presentation. The extra rule on answering questions is that under no circumstances should you answer them. Once you have finished say: "Does that answer your question?" If the questioner has the affrontery to say no, then don't answer his question again – only at greater length. This formula can be repeated if necessary, but a third non-answer is hardly ever needed.

This guide is written, you will have judged, from long experience. I've made all these mistakes – and more. Kurt

Vonnegut boasts that he gave such bad lectures when a lecturer at New York University that he fell asleep during his own lectures. I remember giving a lecture in Manchester on creativity in science where the entire audience was almost unconscious and I suddenly thought: "This is rubbish, utter rubbish". I was tempted to stop and say: "You're not enjoying this and nor am I. Let's stop and go down the pub." I didn't and thank goodness that I didn't – otherwise it wouldn't have been an outstandingly bad presentation.

Summary

- Good presentations resemble each other but bad ones come in many forms

- Lack of preparation, preparing for the wrong audience, making the talk too long or short and ignoring the topic all contribute to a bad presentation

- Visual aids of poor quality, which are too numerous or with too much information, can be a hindrance

- Mumbling, reading from a script and lack of eye contact are all signs of a boring presentation

- A bad presentation rarely produces any questions

10 How to chair a session

ROGER HORTON

Chairing a session at a scientific meeting is like so many things in life – do a good job and no one will notice you or remember your name, but do a bad job and you will be blamed for everything, including the incoherent speaker who left his slides at home. The key to successfully chairing a session is to do your homework thoroughly.

What type of meeting?

The role and responsibilities of the chairman will be coloured by the type of meeting. Often you begin to learn the trade at a small, one-day learned society meeting, by chairing a short session of free communications, delivered by junior colleagues. The venue is probably familiar, the audience small, the atmosphere supportive, and the speakers petrified! A natural progression is to the larger, national conference, spread over several days with parallel sessions, and with a more intense and sometimes adversarial atmosphere.

In attempting to offer advice, I have selected what many would consider the "worst case scenario". The meeting is a large prestigious world congress, held overseas. You have agreed to chair a half-day symposium, comprising six speakers, in an area with which you are familiar, but not an expert. The venue is a conference centre, also using several local hotels, in a city not known to you. You did not organise the symposium and none of the speakers are known to you. International reputations, including yours, may be built and lost in such situations. In dealing with this (unlikely) set of circumstances I will set out the principles and timing which the reader can adapt to less demanding situations.

First principle: get started early

Three months before the meeting

Get to know your speakers and their work. The mechanics are relatively simple these days. As a starting point, search by name one of the bibliographic databases, such as Medline or Pubmed. Print off a list of publications, identify those related to the subject of the meeting, obtain off-prints of the papers, and read them. This should help you establish the standing of the speakers, how long they have worked in this particular field, areas of controversy, and recent advances.

Two months before the meeting

By now the meeting abstracts will be printed and the organisers may well have sent you, as chairman, copies of the abstracts of the speakers in your session. If not, request them, together with mail, telephone and e-mail contacts for the speakers.

Make contact with the speakers, preferably by e-mail. Send contact details and copies of abstracts to all speakers and encourage them to make contact with each other, even to exchange slides (one advantage of PowerPoint is the ability to send slides around the world as e-mail attachments – some people argue it's the only advantage). The purpose of all this electronic interchange is to ensure a coherent programme and prevent each speaker giving essentially the same introduction. In the event of a disagreement, you are the referee.

With more and more speakers using computer-generated slides, it is important to find out from the organisers:

- what formats are being supported (PC, Mac)?
- what presentation packages are being supported (Microsoft PowerPoint)?
- what media are supported (CD, Zip-drive, floppy)?

and to identify which speakers will use computer graphics and ensure that they understand the preferred formats. It is worth encouraging the speakers to bring their laptops, complete with software packages and presentations; if things do go wrong, they can always do another down-load of the images.

At this stage you need to ensure that all participants are absolutely clear about the venue and date of the symposium and, above all, the duration of their contribution (for example, 25 minutes allowed to speak and 10 minutes for questions). Ask speakers to arrive 15 minutes before the start of the session for a briefing. It is also good at this point to ask contributors for copies of papers in press. This avoids any surprises at a later date.

You also need to establish any special requirements such as dual projection or video and to relay this information to the meeting secretariat.

If circumstances allow, I try to organise a social event for the speakers on the day before the session. This may be just meeting for coffee in the conference centre or going out for a meal. This is particularly valued by junior speakers who can be overawed by speaking on the same programme as "superstars". It is helpful to get agreement for this before the meeting. The local organisers will usually suggest appropriate venues and may even make bookings.

One to two days before the session

Venue-related

Make an effort to attend other sessions in the same venue. It is important that you, as chairman, are clear about the technical aspects of the arrangements and are able to inform the speakers authoritatively. It also gives you an opportunity to learn from other people's mistakes.

What should I be looking for?

- Are microphones necessary for speakers? Are they podium-mounted or attached to the speaker?
- Can speakers be clearly heard? Sit in different parts of the auditorium to find out.
- Do speakers control the slides or do they ask a technician to do so?
- Do the technicians have a good command of the English language; in particular, do they understand focus, go back one slide, next slide?
- Do the arrangements work well for conventional slides and computer graphics? They have to, because there is nothing more disastrous for a meeting than major foul-ups with slides.
- Do members of the audience need to use microphones when asking questions? Are there sufficient numbers? Are they easily identified?

- Can the platform and the audience hear the questions?
- Is the venue easy to find and well signposted?
- Is there a technician present throughout? If not, how can one be contacted in an emergency?
- Is the room a comfortable temperature and adequately ventilated?

Some might regard the above as unnecessary, over-fussy, and not the responsibility of the chairman. However, it is clear that if you are able to identify potential problems in advance you have a chance of fixing them; if you find out on the day, you have no chance.

Speaker-related

One of the greatest anxieties of chairing a meeting, particularly if you are also an organiser, is: will the speakers actually show up?

Checking with the meeting secretariat that the speakers have registered (and therefore arrived) can help to allay these fears. At the same time, you can obtain details of their local accommodation to confirm the time and venue of any social function and of the meeting.

Remind speakers to arrive 15 minutes before the session is due to start for a briefing.

On the day

Arrive at least half an hour before the session is due to start.

- Make sure any notices are displayed.
- Make yourself known to the audio-visual technician and ensure slides have been handed in from all speakers (it is now usual for this to be done the day before for morning sessions or early morning for afternoon sessions). Check that they are clearly labelled, have been checked for correct orientation, and do not jam in the projector. Ensure that any computer-generated graphics have been checked. Ensure that the technician knows the running order.
- Check that any special requirements, for example video, are in place.
- Check the sound and the laser pointer (have a spare laser pointer about your person).
- Check that there is an adequate supply of water and clean glasses.
- It can be helpful to the audience to display a slide or overhead with the title of the session. How many times have you found yourself sitting in the wrong room?

- Hold a briefing session for speakers 15 minutes before the session is due to start. This should include: introductions for any participants who have not previously met; making technical arrangements for slides, graphics, sound, and lights; reiterating the timing and advising speakers on how you will indicate when they have five minutes left, and when their time is up (visual cues are often the best); having a reassuring word with the junior and less experienced speakers; and attending to bodily functions – you may be in the room for two hours.

So at last you are all set to go.

- Start the session on time. If you are unable to keep to time, don't expect your speakers to do so.
- Introduce yourself and any co-chairman, welcome the audience and outline any housekeeping details (coffee breaks, meals, etc). Sometimes the chairman gives a brief introduction to the session. Make it brief.
- Introduce the presentations by title and by speaker.
- Ensure that the speakers stick to time. An over-run of one or two minutes into a five-minute discussion session or three minutes into a ten-minute discussion session is the maximum that should be allowed.

If speakers ignore your visual cues, you must interrupt, politely but firmly, requesting the speakers to conclude their presentations. It is very unprofessional and discourteous for speakers to over-run. They are effectively saying that what I have to say is more important than what the other speakers have to say. It is your job to prevent this. At the end of each presentation, thank the speaker and request questions or comments. Identify those wishing to ask questions and request that they identify themselves and their affiliation. Ensure that the audience are able to hear the question and repeat the question if necessary.

- Encourage brief questions – do not allow the questioner to give a lecture.
- Encourage brief answers – do not allow the speaker to give another lecture.
- Try to ensure that all questioners get an opportunity (time permitting). If time runs out, make a mental note of who was unable to ask their questions and try to give them an opportunity to ask questions later.

- Ensure that one or two individuals do not hog the questioning.
- If the discussion gets too heated, then it is your job to cool it down with a diplomatic intervention.
- Ensure that you always have one or two questions ready should the audience be stunned into silence. This is unusual but it does happen, and a little forward planning prevents embarrassment for the speaker and the chairman.
- Keep to time. Curtailment of coffee and lunch breaks to catch up is invariably unpopular with catering staff and the audience.

At the end of the session

- Publicly thank speakers, organisers, sponsors, and audience. A private word of thanks to each of the speakers and to technical staff is usually greatly appreciated.
- Congratulate yourself on a job well done (no one else will) and enjoy the rest of the meeting.

Summary

- The key to successfully chairing a session is to do your homework thoroughly

- The role and responsibilities of the chair will be coloured by the type of meeting

- Get to know your speakers and their work a few months before the meeting

- Identify what visual aids the speakers will be using and familiarise yourself with the technical arrangements of the venue

- On the day of the session, get there early to check that everything is organised and running to schedule

- Ensure that the speakers keep to their allotted time

Index